NOT WITHOUT A
FIGHT

Donna Redman

Order this book online at www.trafford.com
or email orders@trafford.com

Most Trafford titles are also available at major online book retailers.

Printed in the United States of America.

ISBN: 978-1-4669-9384-6 (sc)
ISBN: 978-1-4669-9383-9 (hc)
ISBN: 978-1-4669-9382-2 (e)

Library of Congress Control Number: 2013908943

Trafford rev. 05/17/2013

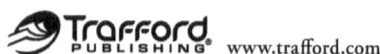

www.trafford.com

North America & international
toll-free: 1 888 232 4444 (USA & Canada)
phone: 250 383 6864 ✦ fax: 812 355 4082

The ultimate value of illness is that it teaches us the value of being alive . . . Death is no enemy of life; it restores our sense of the value of living . . . To learn more about value and proportion we need to honor illness, and ultimately to honor death.

—Arthur Frank,
At the Will of the Body: Reflections on Illness
(Houghton Mifflin)

Acknowledgements

This book would not have been possible without my dear friend Eloisa Bergere Brown. As a writer/journalist, she advised Tammy and me to save all e-mails and correspondence relating to Tammy's illness and to take notes and keep journals, just in case we might need them someday. Then she loaned us her laptop computer to take with us on our adventures. She has offered her insight and encouragement throughout the book writing process.

Charlotte Whaley, who had been a writer and publisher, offered invaluable suggestions. Isabel Sanchez, my editor at the Albuquerque Journal, had the courage to tell me when I wandered off on the wrong track. My uncle, Charles Towner, offered financial help when we needed it. So many people offered insight and suggestions, and my gratitude goes to all of them.

Finally I want to thank my family, including daughters Terri and Cindy and my late husband, Wayne, for their endless support and love.

-1-

March 2003

$\mathcal{I}$ feel compelled to go through Tammy's things over and over again, to touch and smell the things she lived in and with. Each object, whether it's an earring or a book or a sweater, still holds the essence of her, and I want to hold her essence just a little while longer. I don't want time to steal it from me.

Here is one of her trophies—Lokahi Canoe Club, Most Inspirational Crew, 1987. She was a senior at the University of Hawaii that year. She and Terri were seniors in high school when we moved to Hawaii. Wayne (their dad and my husband) worked for the US Department of Agriculture, and in those days, if he wanted a promotion, he had to accept a transfer every couple of years or so. By the time Tammy and Terri graduated, they had attended three different high schools in three states. Their older sister, Cindy, was tired of moving when Wayne transferred to Honolulu, so she stayed behind in San Antonio, Texas, to work on her bachelor's degree at the university there.

Though most of the kids in the Ts' classes at McKinley High in Waikiki were very short Orientals and the Ts were very tall—nearly six feet tall—Tammy and Terri got along just fine. Their buddies called them the Redman Trees and quickly introduced them to island ways. For example, the Ts played clarinet in the marching band, and after football games, everybody went for saimin instead of hamburgers or hot dogs. And everybody hung out at the beach instead of fast-food joints. In short order, both girls learned to bodysurf and to paddle an outrigger canoe.

Terri and Tam are mirror-image identical twins, so Terri, the oldest by one whole minute, is left-handed, while Tammy was right-handed. They loathed being referred to as the twins, but they didn't mind at all being called the Ts. Each struggled to find and maintain her own identity, separate from the other, yet they both liked the same things, had the same friends, and wanted to do the same things at the same time. Maintaining the peace could get a bit tricky at times.

When they were babies, Terri and Tam seemed to need to touch each other before they could go to sleep. They both slept in the same crib, crossways instead of lengthwise. Later, they learned to sleep in separate cribs, but they still needed to be able to see each other before they could relax. By the time they earned their bachelor's degrees, they were determined to finally go their separate ways.

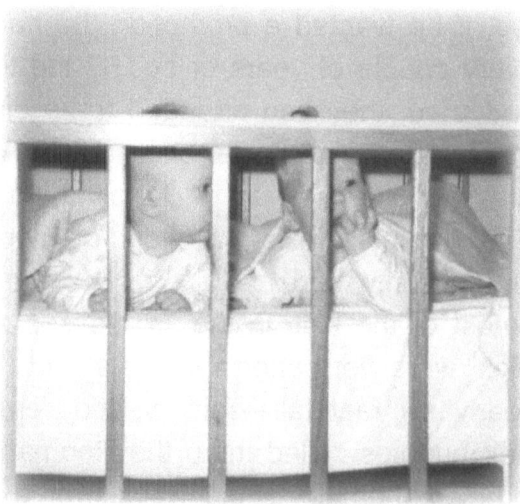

Two babies in a crib—Tammy and Terri,
at about four months, lounging in their crib.

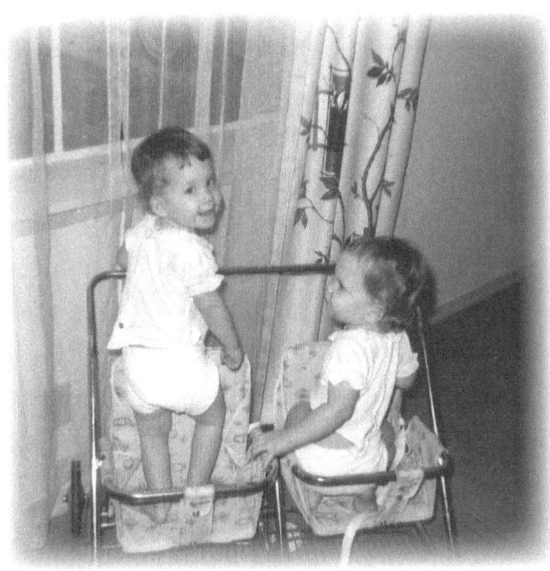

Tammy and Terri, about a year old, getting into mischief.

Here's a second-place trophy for the Brookwood Run 10K in 1993. Tam lived in Birmingham, Alabama, then. She had come to Albuquerque from Hawaii to attend graduate school at the University of New Mexico. When her program was downsized, she transferred to the University of Alabama at Birmingham, where she earned her PhD in microbiology in 1995.

Here are several trophies and medals from her Birmingham days. This one is a participation medal for a marathon. I didn't know she ever ran a marathon.

The medals are wrapped in a red T-shirt she got for participating in a 10K run in Hawaii in 1983. Oh, and here, underneath several pairs of shorts, is a small chess set with quartz chess pieces. I had no idea she played chess. She must have learned in Birmingham.

At the very bottom of the box, there are a couple of Christmas tree ornaments. One is a tiny wooden lobster, and the other is a tiny mandolin. Nothing ordinary for my Tammy!

There are yet more boxes. Those with clothing have other things tucked in them too. This one has a small wicker box with a lid on it. The box is about four inches across, and inside there are all sorts of odds and ends—a pair of earrings made to look like tiny evergreen wreaths, another pair of small round glass Christmas tree ornament earrings, a bottle-cap opener, a small Swiss Army knife, a motley assortment of key rings, and a tiny pair of scissors.

There are boxes and boxes of papers, each with folders labeled and filed alphabetically. Most of them are about things I've never heard of before, probably information she collected while she was in graduate school. And then there are the files about cancer. I don't want to look at those. I put the lid back on the box and put it away.

Tammy has an eclectic collection of books: James Michener's *Hawaii*, several books by Arthur Clarke and Robert Heinlein, and even a collection of Shakespeare's works. Here's Viktor Frankl's *Man's Search for Meaning*, the *National Geographic Photography Field Guide*, *Cats of the World*, and *All I Need to Know I Learned from My Cat*. My curious daughter pursued information about all sorts of things, it seems.

All these CDs, and to think these are what's left after she sold most of her collection to get some much-needed cash. I remember this one by Mary Chapin Carpenter. Tam's favorite track was "The Bug", especially the part that said "Sometimes you're the windshield, sometimes You're the Bug".

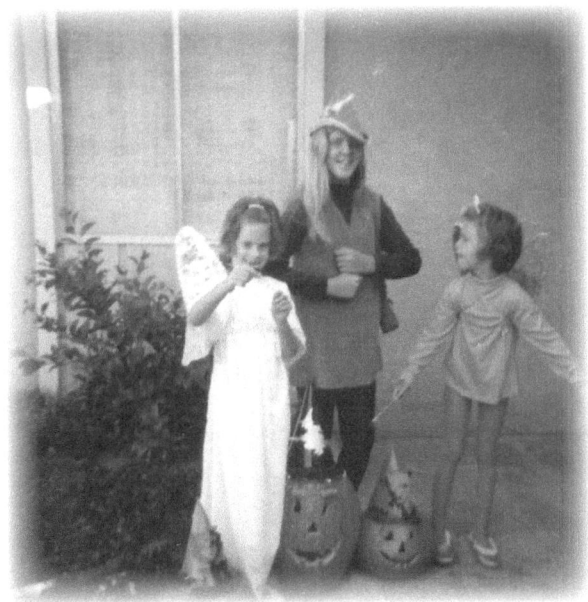

Terri, Cindy and Tammy ready for Halloween festivities. Terri and Tam both wanted to wear wings, but they absolutely did not want to dress up alike. This was the compromise; Terri went as an angel, Tammy dressed up as a fairy.

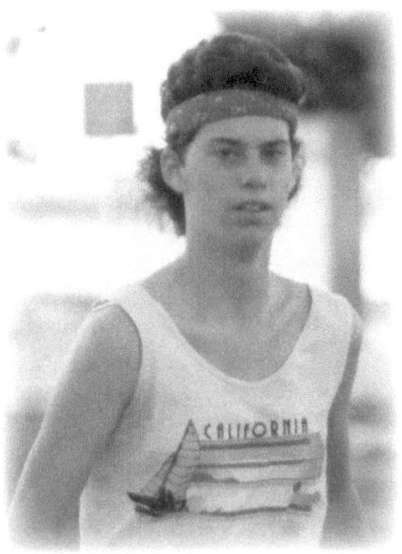

Tammy finishing a competitive run.

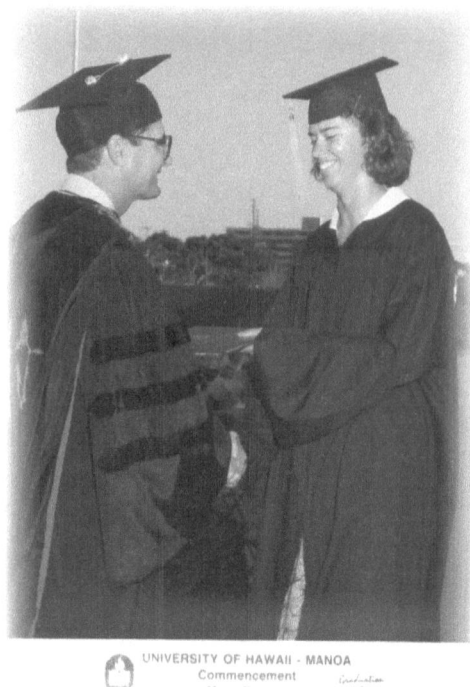

UNIVERSITY OF HAWAII - MANOA
Commencement
May 17 1987

Tammy receiving her diploma at her graduation
from the University of Hawaii.

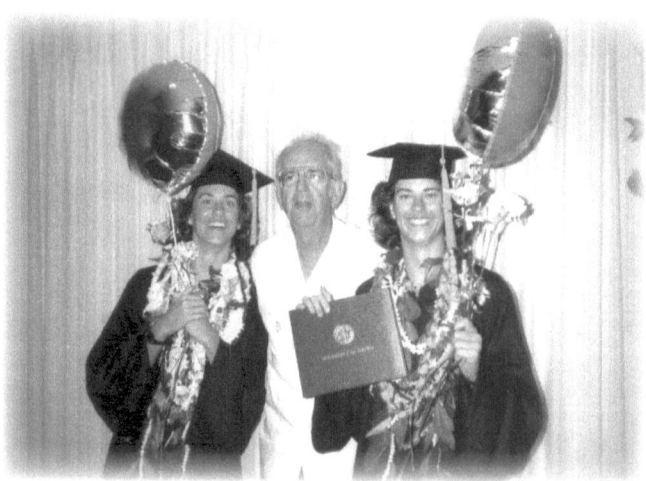

Terri, her Dad, Wayne and Tammy celebrate after the Ts
graduation from the University of Hawaii.

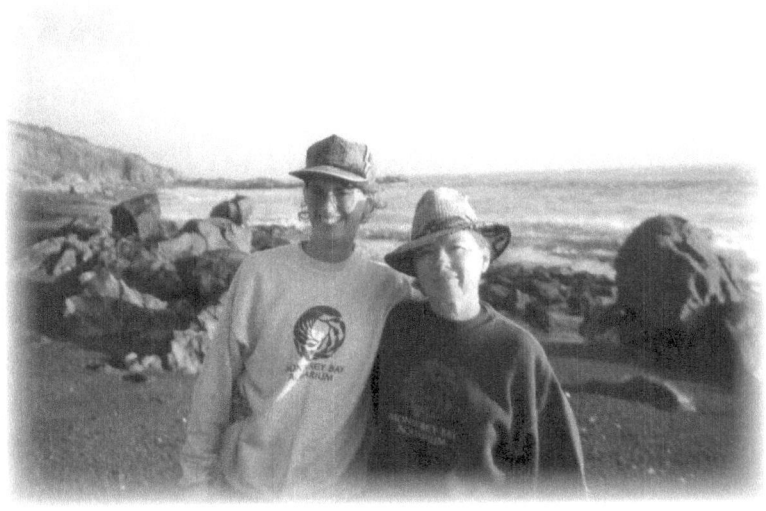

Tammy and her mom, the author, on the beach.

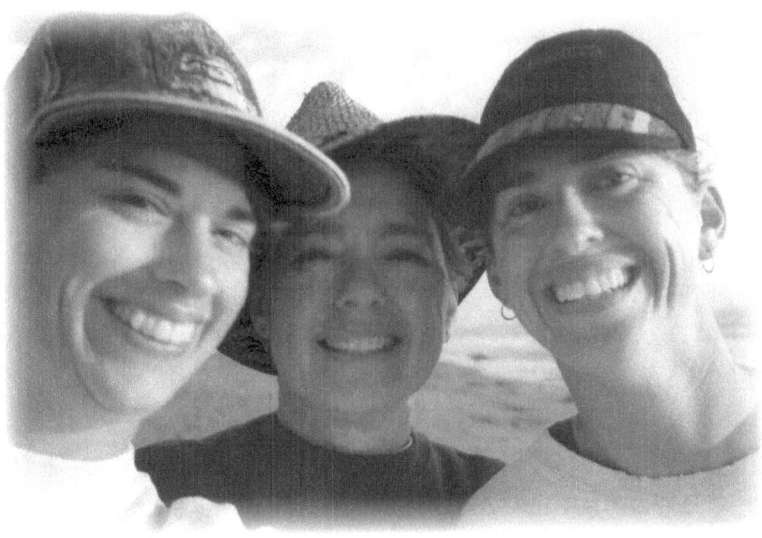

Tammy, the author and Terri with the beach in the background.

-2-

Our family scattered across the country once all three of our daughters were grown. Tammy started graduate school at the University of New Mexico in Albuquerque. Terri went to graduate school at the University of Miami in Florida, and their older sister, Cindy, lived with her husband and two young daughters in San Antonio, Texas. Wayne and I lived in Hawaii. When he retired from the US Department of Agriculture in 1987, we moved to Albuquerque to be near our parents and siblings in Arizona and still be within driving distance of our girls.

A year after our move, Tammy transferred to the University of Alabama at Birmingham to finish her PhD in microbiology. Meanwhile, within a couple of years, both Terri and Cindy and her family had moved to Albuquerque.

After she finished her PhD, Tammy continued working as a postdoctoral fellow in Birmingham. Though she worked long hours, she was diligent about keeping up with what was going on with the rest of the family and letting us know what was going on with her.

"Hey, Terri," she said during one of her regular phone calls. "I've been thinking about this a lot lately. With all the money I spend on phone calls and trips home to see you guys, I think it would be much cheaper and better all around for me if I just move back to Albuquerque. I shouldn't have any trouble finding a job there. What do you think?"

The year was 1997.

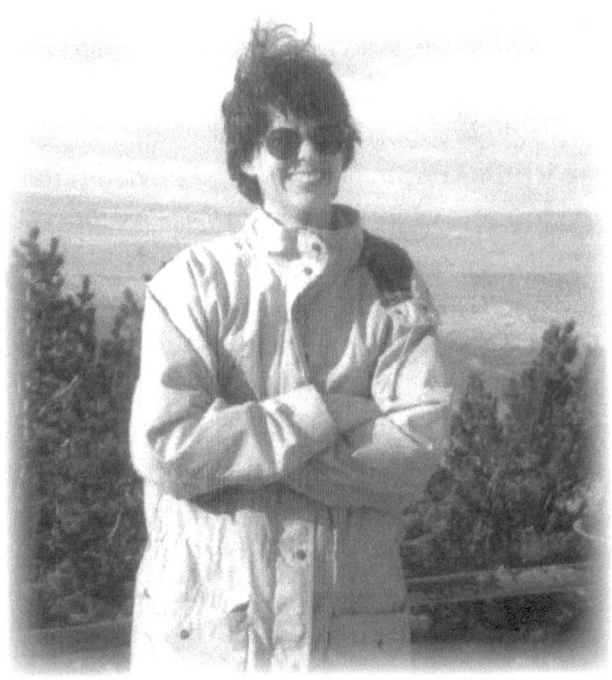

Tammy at the crest of Sandia Mountain, east of Albuquerque.

Overjoyed, Terri bought an old—over fifty-year-old—house near the University of New Mexico campus for her and Tam to share. Tammy paid rent, but as far as each of them was concerned, the house belonged to them both.

The house had been a rental for years, and it was run-down, but it was in one of those old-fashioned neighborhoods where everybody knew everybody else. All the neighbors got together for picnics in the park down the street on the Fourth of July. They exchanged small gifts at Christmastime. They brought food if someone was sick. And they were seldom too busy to stop and chat.

Terri and Tammy loved the neighborhood, and they loved the old house.

They painted and repaired and updated it until it was their own. They turned the badly neglected yard into a green refuge.

They both loved plants in general and gardening in particular, and their yard showed it. They trimmed and fed and coddled the row of ancient rosebushes along one side of their front yard. They hauled out trash, and they cut down the dead cottonwood tree in the backyard. They contoured and they planted. One side of the backyard had apparently been a vegetable garden, so they cleaned it out and planted their vegetables there. But not in neat straight rows—that would be too regimented, too ordinary for them. The tomatoes were planted in a cluster, and the cucumbers wound around at their feet. So it went with the rest of the garden: two rows of flowers, one yellow calendulas and the other bright blue lobelia, twisted and turned in the shape of a double helix throughout the vegetable garden. Sunflowers lined the sidewall.

Terri and Tammy spent hours sitting in the cool shade in their backyard, just watching things grow. I had my doubts when they decided to live together. True, they were best friends. They even had their own twin-speak, as many twins do—they made it up first even before they learned to talk so the rest of the world could understand what they were saying. They were both fanatic about exercise, especially swimming and running and cycling. But Terri was like a Super Ball, always in motion, always in a hurry, while Tammy moved at a much slower pace. She was more methodical, more laid-back. Terri was a neatnik, while Tammy was a bit messy sometimes. I was worried about them getting along together in one house again after living apart for so many years.

But they got along just fine.

Then, in 1998, Tammy was diagnosed with cancer.

Nine years earlier, almost to the day, I had been diagnosed with leiomyosarcoma, a fast-growing type of cancer that attacks smooth muscles. But I was fortunate because my tumor was growing on the lining of the common femoral vein in my left groin, and it made its presence known early on. It made my left leg swell, and the search for the cause of the swelling led to the discovery of a golf-ball-sized tumor.

It was surgically removed, and when the biopsy confirmed the diagnosis of cancer, my doctors rushed me through a series of scans and tests and started my treatment right away.

At first I was angry—not at anyone or anything specifically, but just generally angry. The first time I went to the oncologist's office and saw a partially completed jigsaw puzzle on a coffee table in the waiting room, I saw that as an ominous sign that somebody expected me to be spending a whole lot of time in that waiting room, and I was not pleased.

I was absolutely obsessed with maintaining the status quo; I was not going to let cancer control my life. But when my hair started coming out in clumps and I ended up bald, my anger turned to bewilderment and sorrow and a reevaluation of my priorities.

After three sessions of chemotherapy (one a month), I had a series of radiation treatments followed by three more chemo sessions. During the interruption in chemo while I had radiation, my hair had come back curly (it's naturally straight—this was a great bonus!), but when I started the final session of chemo treatments, my hair fell out again. This time it wasn't such a shock. And I came to actually enjoy playing with those jigsaw puzzles in my oncologist's office by the time all my treatments were finished.

I had all sorts of scans and tests on a regular basis after I finished the treatment regimen. Each time, I expected dire results, but each time, there was no sign of the cancer. I just knew every strange bump and each unexplained ache or pain meant that the cancer was back, but it never was. Long after I was declared cancer-free, I still expected it to pop back up again. But eventually I came to believe that maybe it really was over.

In retrospect, I see that I was extraordinarily lucky. My tumor was found early, before it spread. Tammy wasn't so lucky. She was diagnosed with cancer, angiosarcoma, on the same leg, only hers was on her buttock. I saw my oncologist in a restaurant not long after Tammy's diagnosis, and I told her about Tammy.

"Oh my gosh!" she said. "Did you know your diagnosis was changed from leiomyosarcoma to angiosarcoma? Your daughter has the same cancer you had, and it's a really, really rare one."

After a while, Tammy started keeping a journal of her cancer odyssey, detailing events as well as her impressions of what was going on now that her life revolved around cancer. At first she didn't post entry dates; she just wrote what was on her mind.

This is what she had to say about her first encounter with cancer, with hash marks marking the end of each entry:

"Hey, is there a bump on my butt?"
In the beginning I thought it was an innocuous bug bite or a splinter. I asked Terri to inspect the back of my left thigh.
"I don't see anything," she said.
Jokingly, I responded in a lame impersonation of Arnold Schwarzenegger, "It's probably just a tumah on my ahss."
Several months later, it turned out that I truly did have a tumor on my butt. It wasn't funny.

I first noticed the bump on the back of my leg in November 1997 after helping Cindy clear weeds out of her backyard. At the end of November, I went to see my doctor about the bump. She thought it may be an abscess and prescribed antibiotics. I took the antibiotics and went on with my life.

In March, I noticed that the damned bump was still there, so I went back to the doc. She said that sometimes the infected tissue gets walled off from the healthy tissue and the resulting bump can last for months. She decided to try to do a needle aspiration. The bump was solid—nothing came out. So I got more antibiotics and went on my way.

Now the bump began changing. It grew larger, and the surface grew flat and red, and it began to feel warm to the touch. I went back a third time to the doctor. She said she had never seen anything like it, and she felt strongly that it needed to be removed. She said that another physician in her practice was more experienced at these small in-office procedures.

He thought it was probably a benign lipoma, and later that afternoon, he removed an ugly mass from my buttock. A nurse carefully cleaned and tightly bandaged the wound, and I went home.

The next day, I felt pressure building under the skin where the "lipoma" had been removed, and later in the afternoon, the wound opened up and began bleeding again. I went back to see the doctor, and he drained as much blood as he could and reapplied the bandaging.

I went back to the doctor every day that week. By the weekend, it looked like the wound might be healing. But when I took a shower Saturday evening, I saw a trickle of blood from my leg. It soon turned to a horrifying river of blood. I screamed for Terri—thank God for a sister who's a physical therapist with training in wound treatment.

She calmly helped me out of the shower and stopped the bleeding, then bandaged me up.

Monday morning, I called the doctor about my recurrent bleeding problem. He agreed that something needed to be done, so he referred me to a general surgeon. The next Wednesday, Mom and I went to see him.

Meanwhile, the pathology report finally came back saying the mass was a benign hemangioendothelioma.

When I saw the surgeon, he ordered a CT scan before he scheduled surgery to remove the mass, which was rapidly growing back. The scan showed it localized to the fat just under the skin of my buttock.

The surgery was no problem. I went home with some stitches to be removed by a physician's assistant in a couple of weeks.

Just a few days later, someone from the surgeon's office called saying I needed to come back and speak directly with the surgeon. That's when I knew the mass was not benign.

My life moved in very slow motion, but time sped by. I left my office and went for a two-hour walk in the desert to try and sort out my thoughts.

I realized I knew nothing about the kind of cancer I had or the treatment options. So I decided to focus on my immediate comfort.

It was June in New Mexico, and my car's air conditioner didn't work. I figured it was going to be a rough summer, and I wanted to at least have a comfortable car to ride in. My car, a stunning, classic old Saab, was getting expensive to maintain. I decided to trade it in and get a brand-new Subaru Impreza Outback Sport. That afternoon I looked at some—and drove one home. I bought the car on absolutely blind faith that somehow things would work out and I would be able to keep it.

I met with the surgeon after work last Friday. He told me that I had an angiosarcoma, a rare soft-tissue sarcoma. He said I needed much more extensive surgery to remove any remnants of the tumor.

I also talked to a plastic surgeon. I'm to have a wide excision to remove the lower half of my left buttock and any remaining cancerous cells, followed by reconstructive surgery using tissue from the back of my thigh to fill in the hole. The incision will extend from midbuttock to just above the back of my knee.

I felt numb. I walked out of the clinic feeling so different from everyone else. I went home and took a three-hour walk, trying to get used to the idea that I have cancer.

The surgery took several hours. I barely remember waking up in the hospital. I came home only to fall asleep again. I slept most of the first few days, but I immediately felt that the tumor was gone; the monster draining the life out of me was gone. I could stand on my reconstructed leg immediately after coming home from the hospital, but walking, dressing, and bathing were a little tricky.

Every day I got a little stronger and a little more mobile. After a couple of weeks, I could slowly walk around the block, and after three weeks, I went back to work.

Although the surgery was a success (no cancer cells in the margins of the removed tissue) and I was doing heavy-duty physical therapy, I'm not yet done with treatment.

I still need to have thirty-seven radiation treatments to the back of my leg.

The radiation oncologist asked me if I would be getting chemotherapy. I said that I was told it wasn't necessary. He said he thought I should talk to an oncologist, so I got a referral to one. I began to scour the medical literature for any information about angiosarcoma and about sarcomas in general.

I learned that sarcomas are extremely rare cancers. In 1995 in the United States, only seven thousand sarcoma cases were statistically predicted to be diagnosed, and of those only about seventy were predicted to be angiosarcoma, soft-tissue sarcomas that involve blood vessels. The treatment for angiosarcoma usually consisted of surgery, radiation, and sometimes chemotherapy, depending on the size and location of the tumor.

###

The oncologist feels chemotherapy is unnecessary for me. My tumor is thought to be relatively small (less than five centimeters, or about two inches). (But after I got home, it dawned on me that the oncologist didn't realize that the tumor had been cut on three times, so it was impossible to determine the original size.) However, since my tumor is close to the surface of the skin and not in any organs, they feel that the risks of chemotherapy outweigh the advantages. The chances of a recurrence are about fifty-fifty, and chemotherapy won't change those odds. However, radiation therapy is necessary.

I pretty much sailed through the radiation, except that I got so tired. At first it really wasn't too bad. I went to work until 3:30 p.m., then I went for radiation treatments. As my skin got more and more burned, I began swimming after the treatments. The nurses didn't approve of this at all, but the doc said that if I was careful not to wipe off the radiation markings, it would be okay. So I slathered my leg with Vaseline and got in the soothing pool. I'm convinced that swimming helped.

After swimming I was completely exhausted. The exhaustion hit me every day about four hours after treatment, and after four weeks of treatments, I was just exhausted all the time. It took about six months to really start feeling like my old self again. The seven-and-a-half weeks of treatment were absolutely grueling, but time went by and I got through it.

However, the quality and quantity of my work suffered because I wasn't able to work forty-five—to fifty-hour weeks like my counterparts. I worked as a postdoctoral fellow at a lung biology research facility where I studied respiratory immunology as a PhD microbiologist. During the roughly five months of surgeries and treatments, I wasn't able to do enough to get promoted to a regular staff scientist position.

Frankly, my heart just isn't in it anymore.

###

I'm regaining function in my leg. I'm on a follow-up schedule where I receive CTs and MRIs every three months. First one follow-up and then another and then another have gone by. It looks like the cancer is really gone. But it's still difficult for me to think about the future.

I'm working to reclaim my body from the wreckage brought on by the cancer. At first I could barely walk around the block, but I did it anyway. I worked first with a physical therapist, then an exercise physiologist. I swam regularly and exercised both at a gym and at home until I could finally walk without a limp. My plastic surgeon didn't think I ever would, but I can.

But I feel betrayed by my body, the body that I've always tried to take such good care of. I feel guilty because I must have done something to cause the cancer. I feel angry because I'm trying to become established as a scientist but I can't work as hard or be as productive during my treatments as before my cancer. But most of all, I feel helpless, completely out of control of my life.

While I was lying on the couch, waiting to heal, I decided to be a survivor.

I've heard people say that having cancer has been a blessing for them because it has given them a chance to get their lives in order. I don't believe cancer is a blessing or a curse—it just happens. And it's really, really tragic because it impacts way more than the one fighting it. Family and friends, all the people who truly care for the cancer patient, are deeply affected too.

I'm going to a counselor now and taking antidepressant medication. I've always been a little on the depressed side; having cancer really exaggerates it. Dealing with cancer treatment and the realization of your own mortality affects every part of your life and amplifies any problems or fears that you had to deal with before getting sick.

After all her treatments were finished and it looked like her cancer had been eradicated, Tammy seemed to feel she had a debt to repay—a debt for her survival, a debt to all those who didn't survive.

When I finished my cancer treatments, I didn't ever want to say or hear the word "cancer" again. I felt that by some miracle or fluke, I had escaped the wrath of cancer; I didn't want to draw its attention to me again. I steadfastly avoided support groups and their ilk. But not Tammy. She was determined to declare war on the monster and face it head-on. She joined a cancer support group, not so much to get support as to give it. She volunteered to do computer work for the breast cancer information center at her HMO (health maintenance organization).

Though she was still vitally interested in pursuing the mysteries of science, her primary focus seemed to shift from building a career to helping others beat cancer too. She was determined to ferret out all the information she could find about surviving this monstrosity.

Her mind was wide open, unhindered by bias for or against any particular avenue to recovery, whether it was conventional medicine or an alternative. However, she was armed with a determined skepticism. She wanted proof before she embraced any regimen.

As time went on, it became more and more difficult for her to work in a career that required her to make long-term plans for the future. She couldn't make long-term plans for her own future, because she still didn't know if she truly had one.

From Tammy's journal:

I don't want to work as a postdoctoral fellow anymore. I need to do something that has more immediate satisfaction and more personal interactions than being holed up at a desk all day writing papers and proposals.

At first I had no idea what, other than biomedical research, I could possibly do. I thought about going to medical school or physician's assistant school or dental school. I was repeating the same kind of behavior that motivated me to earn a PhD. I felt that I didn't have the skills to get a job and support myself.

What I actually lack is self-confidence or even an awareness of what I have to offer. I thought school was the answer to my problems. I'm very good at learning. I know I could succeed in some kind of educational program.

But I just can't afford to go back to school. I began reading classified ads in the paper as well as on biomedical-related web pages. I answered several ads, including those advertising jobs for pharmaceutical sales reps, public health and education positions, and science writing jobs. Finally, I got an interesting offer from a company in Boston that's working on developing an online database of information gleaned from research literature. Proteome is looking for people with PhDs in science to read scientific papers, identify the salient information, summarize that information using a controlled vocabulary, and enter the information into the database. What's more, Proteome will do on-the-job training.

This is just what I'm looking for.

I accepted the Proteome job and went to Boston for a weekend of training, then began working as a scientific curator. This allowed me to quit the postdoctoral-fellow job and gave me time to decide what I want to do with the rest of my life. Through the COBRA Program, I can pay the premiums and keep my health insurance in force.

The Proteome job turned out to be trickier than I anticipated, but I view it as a challenge, so I'm going to keep at it. I enjoy reading the papers, but it's tough looking at a computer screen for hours on end, all alone. While it was a relief to get away from laboratory work, I'm starting to feel isolated. So I applied for a part-time teaching position at Albuquerque Technical Vocational Institute (TVI), a local community college.

I'm teaching two sections of an introductory biology lab for students interested in pursuing careers in allied health— nursing, respiratory therapy, operating room assistants, etc.

I enjoy teaching the laboratory classes, and I enjoy getting to know each of the students and their backgrounds and goals. To improve my teaching skills, I'm taking an instructor's development class offered by TVI. I find it fascinating. This is a place where I can have positive, effective, and challenging interactions with other people. And even though I don't have formal training as a teacher, I can do a good job here.

At the end of the term, it was devastating to read some of the student evaluations. I felt they were unfair and harsh. But after talking to other instructors, I learned that students who do poorly tend to write unpleasant evaluations. It was also interesting that several of the students perceived my inability to answer some of their questions as a lack of confidence, when actually I had no qualms about admitting when I simply didn't know.

The second term is going very well. I'm delighted to be making more money than ever before by working two part-time jobs. It's a good balance. Life is good, my follow-up scans so far are clear, and I can put the cancer behind me and begin thinking of it as a minor roadblock. What's more, I actually find myself thinking about the future as if I just might have one, after all.

###

Tammy loved the freedom to work on the computer whenever she felt like it. She could work in her pajamas if she wanted or work in the middle of the night if she was having trouble sleeping. From where she sat at her computer, she could look out and watch the young desert willow tree and the small patch of lavender plants grow. With the French doors open, she could smell the sage and the rosemary. She could see the sunflowers and the penstemons and the trumpet vine twining up the fence at the back of the yard. She and Terri had hung bird feeders from the back porch, and she watched the hummingbirds, the finches, and the LBJs (little brown jobs, the birds they couldn't identify) as they fed and bustled around the yard. It all brought her a sense of peace, I think.

Richard lived across the street. Tammy met him when she was working to regain full use of her left leg after the surgery. He was a Rolfer, a therapist who used systematic massaging of the deep muscles to help Tammy regain strength in her leg. He was certain that he could help her, and he did.

He was taller than Tammy, probably 6'1" or 6'2", and lean. He was perhaps ten or fifteen years older than Tam and had a full head of unruly white hair, with a tiny eight-inch-long braid at the bottom in back, his tribute to the latent hippie in his soul.

He was the divorced father of a seven-year-old son and a ten-year-old daughter, and he had moved to the neighborhood to be near his children. His son had leukemia. Tammy agreed to help Richard write a book about the impact his son's cancer had on the family.

They spent long hours together, talking and laughing—and crying too, I suppose. Sometimes one or both of his children came with him to play with Tammy's and Terri's cats or to explore the backyard and the vegetable garden. Corinna, his daughter, especially liked searching out and harvesting the long pale-green Armenian cucumbers.

Once Tammy regained the full use of her leg, she began riding her bike again. At first she rode short distances, and then she gradually worked up to long rides. Once she could handle long rides, she rejoined a group of her friends—Chris Glidden and Chris's teenage daughter Jenna, Michael Giudicissi, and sometimes Terri—for a three- to four-hour ride every Sunday, no matter what the weather was. (Terri belonged to a different group of cyclists, but occasionally she rode with Tammy's group once Tam started riding again.)

"It was like clockwork for us," Chris told me later.

Sometimes after their ride, the whole group would go back to the Gliddens' home where Chris's husband, Jim, cooked breakfast for them.

Tammy loved living in the old house, and she loved the yard; she loved her new jobs and the freedom they gave her. She loved living with Terri and living near the rest of us, and she loved her neighbors, most especially Richard. For the first time in a very long time, she was content with her life. After her brush with cancer, that happiness was sweet indeed.

-3-

$\mathcal{I}$n July 2001, during a regular checkup, the MRI showed suspicious masses in Tammy's tailbone and up into her spine.

"This doesn't look good," her oncologist said. "This really doesn't look good."

That was the understatement of the decade, but neither Tammy nor I believed it at the time.

Since nobody she talked with in Albuquerque seemed to know much about angiosarcoma, Tammy thought she could do a bit of research and find her own solution to her problem. And I, proud mother that I was, had no doubt that she could do it.

She went along with the usual tests to determine if this was truly a return of her original cancer or something else entirely. Deep down inside she knew that her cancer was back, but her doctors did not, so she agreed to all the poking and prodding and scanning.

The first time around, Tammy's angiosarcoma had been bloody, and it had grown very, very fast. However, it didn't *look* like a malignant tumor.

This time, when the doctor ordered a biopsy, the biopsy seemed to infuriate the tumor in her tailbone—it began to hurt intensely and constantly.

I remember hanging up the phone after Tam called with the results of her biopsy. I remember hearing her tell me the news matter-of-factly as though she were giving me the latest weather report. And I remember responding in kind, then hanging up the phone and sobbing. Finally I dried my eyes and told Wayne that Tam's cancer was back.

"This time we're going to lose her," I said. He took the news quietly. His eyes filled with tears as he put his arms around me and tried to comfort me.

After a while, I shifted from absolute despair to numbness.

Time moved not uniformly but in layers. On one level, it stopped while all the "what if"s and "now what?"s and "dammit, God, this isn't fair!"s swirled around in my mind. On another level, it moved in slow motion. I was detached, watching the events of the day happen, but not really involved. I felt as though I was walking in neck-deep water, and it was very difficult to move at all. And on yet another level, time raced by, with decisions being made and life moving forward too fast for me to keep up. I was going through the motions, but I wasn't actively participating. I was just too numb.

Tam was able to get an appointment to see her oncologist within only a couple of days. Cindy and Terri went with her to see the doctor, both to lend Tam their support and to find out what was happening to her firsthand. Of course I went too.

Only one of us could go in the exam room with her, and she asked me to go with her. I don't know if it was because I'm her mother or because if she chose one of her two sisters, the other would have hurt feelings.

When Tammy asked Dr. Amy Tarnower about the biopsy, she replied, "It was angio [angiosarcoma]. [From the results of the CT and the bone scan] we know it's not in the lungs, we know it's not in the liver. We've got two isolated spots in bone and the spot that you said was hurting you . . . Once it goes outside the original tumor area, it's considered metastatic."

Tammy questioned her to find out exactly where these new tumors were growing, how big they were, and what her options were. Dr. Tarnower answered each question as best she could, but she hadn't had much experience with sarcomas, she said, and none with this particular kind of sarcoma.

One tumor had already destroyed her tailbone; another had nearly consumed the L4 vertebra in her lower back and was moving into L5. Yet another was invading the right sacroiliac joint in her pelvis. Oh, and there was another tumor growing near the original tumor site, at the back of her left thigh.

This was impossible! Just the week before, she had ridden her bicycle seventy miles to raise money for charity. She had just turned thirty-seven. Her whole life was ahead of her.

"This doesn't look good."

Innocuous words, words of doom on that sunny day in July of 2001.

Dr. Tarnower wanted to consult with specialists at the MD Anderson School of Medicine at the University of Texas in Houston and at Harvard's Dana-Farber Cancer Center in Boston, but it might take as long as two weeks to get a response from them, she said.

"A couple of weeks shouldn't make that much difference," she said as she gave Tammy a prescription for pain and sent her home.

"It's ba-ack! And it's in my ba-ack," Tammy told Terri and Cindy when we went back out to the waiting room, trying to make light of the devastating news. "The little bugger ate my tailbone and now it's working its way up my spine, but hey, I'm still walking. Amy doesn't know what to do with it, but somebody somewhere does. We just have to find them."

She laughed as she said it, as though it was a grand joke, but her whole body trembled.

Day by day I could see her slipping, getting sicker and sicker as her disease rapidly progressed. She didn't have "a couple of weeks" to wait!

By the end of that week, Dr. Tarnower had talked to someone at MD Anderson, and the doctor there suggested a short course of Doxil (a chemotherapy drug) to slow the disease progression until they could determine if she would be eligible to participate in one of several clinical trials currently underway. They would try to work her in for a consultation sometime in September, two months away.

Tammy's spine was getting stiffer, and her pain was getting much worse by the hour. If things continued the way they were going, she wouldn't survive until September.

In the meantime, Dr. Tarnower said she could send her to the University of Arizona Cancer Center in Tucson for a consultation, but they couldn't work her in until mid-August.

Tammy thought about that for a while. Then she cried. Then she got mad, really mad. Mad at the situation, mad at the indecision, mad at the delay. She had to do something. So she called Dr. Michael Lobell, the oncologist she was scheduled to see in Tucson, and explained her situation. She told him she could not wait until mid-August for a consultation. He agreed. He scheduled her for a consultation the following week.

Dr. Tarnower started her on the Doxil right away, even before her trek to Tucson. Tam had an appointment to see her after the first round of Doxil, which had been administered intravenously at the cancer center where Dr. Tarnower had her office. She sent the following e-mail before the appointment:

August 1, 2001

Hi Dr. Tarnower,

It's about 10:30 p.m., so you won't be seeing this till tomorrow. Today was blessedly uneventful. The Doxil went very well with no nausea and no headache, just a little fatigue. You hemo./onc. people were jumping today, but you were all very pleasant.

So I'm sending you this little note because I have an outside-of-the-box idea that I would like you to have a chance to think about before we talk again next Tuesday.

One of my mother's friends and my older sister, Cindy, have gotten some information on this place called the Fermilab Midwest Institute for Neutron Therapy. This place is in Illinois, and it's run by a bunch of physicists who were trained to build neutron bombs. Now they are using proton and neutron particle therapy to treat cancer patients, and amazingly, they specifically list angiosarcoma as one tumor that responds very well to the treatment. This treatment involves very high-energy radiation and it's delivered in ten to twelve treatments instead of the thirty to forty treatments with conventional radiation therapy. Apparently this treatment no longer is considered experimental, and the lab treats patients from all over, including MD Anderson. But patients must have a referral. I'm thinking maybe there's just a tiny, tiny chance that after a few rounds of chemo, I could get this treatment and maybe save my spine. I need more info. But that little hope will help me sleep tonight. I'm enclosing some web page information about the institute.

Thanks for your help, and don't give up on me just yet.

Tammy Redman

Dr. Tarnower agreed to research the neutron radiation facility while Tammy was in Tucson.

Terri and Cindy and I went with Tammy to Tucson to lend our moral support, even if we could do nothing else. Because it was the most comfortable vehicle available, we all piled into Terri's brand-new preowned Toyota Rav4 and headed for Tucson. We took all of Tam's pertinent x-rays, films, and test results with us—at least thirty pounds' worth.

-4-

$\mathcal{W}$e had reservations at the Clarion Hotel since they offered special rates for Cancer Center patients and their families. But we couldn't find it. This was before GPS and similar devices were commonly available. We didn't have access to one. We knew the hotel was near the university, but though the street name was familiar, we couldn't even find the street.

It's been a family joke for years that I have absolutely no sense of direction. Consequently everybody feels free to tell me where to go and how to get there, and nobody really listens when I suggest the direction we should be going.

Years ago, we lived in Nogales, Arizona, when Wayne worked on the Mexican border for what was then called the USDA Plant Pest Control. Terri and Tammy were born in Tucson. When we went "to town" to shop or get the car fixed, we went to Tucson. At one time, Tucson was familiar, and even I knew my way around, but no more.

"I think Alvernon Way is closer to the mountains," Cindy said.

"Which mountains?" Terri responded. "There are mountains all around us."

"This way!"

"No, that way."

Aha! They had no better senses of direction than I had! Finally we gave up and bought a map and made our way to the hotel with no more problems. At least we could all read a map. That map proved to be indispensable for all our remaining forays through Tucson.

When we settled into our room, we discovered that it had large sliding glass doors that opened into a small patio. Just beyond the patio, there was a lovely swimming pool. During our entire stay, it was our private pool; no one else seemed to use it.

We spent every spare minute in that pool. All three of my daughters are "water babies," and they did serious lap swimming, even Tammy, just to stretch their travel-weary muscles. I swam a little and puttered around a lot. When they were finished with their workout, they draped their long legs over the edge of the pool and floated on their backs in the water. I tried to join them, but their legs are longer than mine. My body didn't seem to bend in the right places—when I stretched to hook my legs over the edge of the pool, my torso went under the water; it refused to float. When they finally stopped laughing at me, one got on each side of me and held my upper body up on the surface of the water. Eventually I got the hang of it and could do it by myself. We must have looked like a bunch of birds perched on a wire, all four of us in a row, clinging to the pool edge with our legs, floating on our backs in the water.

I can't remember what we talked about. Trivial things, I guess. I know we giggled a lot.

The Arizona Cancer Center is on the campus of the University of Arizona, and it was surprisingly easy to find. The facility was on a lower level, below ground, but there was a large atrium in the center that reached up to open air at the top, so there was sunlight. We expected everybody to be terribly busy, much too busy to bother with us. But everyone we encountered seemed anxious to make Tammy's visit as comfortable and as productive as possible.

First she talked to Dr. Lobell, oncologist and associate professor of clinical medicine at the U of A. Then he arranged to go with her to see oncology radiologist Dr. Dino Stea and finally to see surgeon Dr. James Warneke. It seemed nothing short of miraculous that she was able to see three physicians, all on the same day, with an appointment to see only one of them. It would have taken weeks, if not months, to coordinate schedules to do that with her HMO in Albuquerque.

Tam was armed with all the information she could find about her disease, and she asked endless questions about her treatment options. Since she was a medical research scientist by profession, all the medical jargon made perfect sense to her. She asked technical questions and fully understood the technical answers.

I think she held her tears at bay by focusing on this question-and-answer process. Throughout her medical adventures, she did that. She seemed to step outside herself and become a detached investigator. With doctors who tried to be condescending with her, she put on her "Don't you try to snow me!" attitude to squeeze out every drop of information about her situation. In the process, she intimidated the hell out of some of her doctors, and I thought it was grand; she seemed to think it was no big deal.

She just knew that her prognosis was hers to choose. No matter what the doctors said, her chances couldn't be that grim. She was determined to live.

Dr. Lobell was a small, bent gnome of a man with large feet encased in orthopedic shoes, and after our very first chat with him, he became one of my favorite people in the whole world. He asked question after question, and he listened carefully to Tammy's answers.

In the radiology department waiting room, we watched small iridescent blue and yellow fish dart around their miniature reef in a large saltwater aquarium as we waited to be called to see the doctor. Dr. Dino Stea, the radiation oncologist, was probably in his midforties, and he moved with both energy and grace. He too listened closely to Tammy. He too became one of my favorite people.

When she talked to him about the Neutron Therapy Facility at Fermilab, he said he had heard of it, and it was indeed an effective treatment option. But the expense of travel and lodging, never mind the treatment itself, could be prohibitive.

Finally, Tammy was sent to talk to Dr. James Warneke, an associate professor of surgery and surgical oncology. He was a small, wiry young man who seemed determined to do his best to save Tammy's spine and keep her mobile. During their conversation, Tammy learned that he and his wife enjoyed competitive bicycle riding, just as she did. Yet another good guy.

After Dr. Warneke finished examining her, the other two physicians came into the room, and the three of them talked together and with Tammy about the best treatment options for her. I thought that it was a very good sign indeed that they included her in their discussion.

These three physicians made up a formidable team. Tammy felt that they had the knowledge, the experience, the talent, and the heart to give her a fighting chance for survival.

Perhaps it was because they were her only hope that she trusted their judgment so completely. Or maybe it was because they treated her with dignity, as a real person, not just another disease.

They decided to put Tammy on what Dr. Lobell called hard chemo, a cocktail of high-dose Adriamycin, ifosfamide, and mesna, the latter to protect her bladder from the harsh side effects of the ifosfamide.

"I think that should work very well for you," Dr. Lobell said. "I have an angiosarcoma patient who had much more disease activity than you have who is now in remission after doing that chemo."

First she would have a catheter implanted in her chest so she could have the chemo delivered to her system around-the-clock. And as a bonus, she could also have blood drawn through the catheter for various tests without having to have a needle stuck in her.

She would get several sessions of chemo, and after the chemo, she would have radiation.

"You understand the radiation would be for palliation," Dr. Stea said.

Tammy nodded, and I thought, *Well, sure, whatever the hell palliation is. Just do it!* Later, when I looked it up in the dictionary, I saw that *palliation* means "to alleviate pain." But the neutron radiation offered more, didn't it? It could kill the tumors.

Once the chemotherapy and radiation were finished, she would have surgery to stabilize her spine.

The surgery to insert the catheter, the chemotherapy, and the radiation would be done in Albuquerque unless she could arrange to go to the Neutron Therapy Facility in Illinois for radiation. But she would return to Tucson for the surgery to stabilize her spine.

"We can't give you any guarantees," Dr. Lobell said, "but we can give you hope."

That's all we wanted; that's what we came for.

-5-

We came home from Tucson on a Tuesday, and Tam was scheduled to get her catheter implanted on Friday. As I waited for her to come out of the implant surgery, I felt sorrow—no longer a sharp pain but deep, deep sadness. What happened to yesterday's hope? There were so many mundane details to contend with. Maybe that was a good thing. I shoved the sorrow to the back and focused on the details—little things, like where was the money coming from to pay Tammy's bills if she couldn't work? I wanted to say "Don't worry, we'll take care of it," but our resources were getting awfully, awfully thin. *Keep the faith, things will work out,* I told myself. And I tried; I really tried. But I was so tired, so bone-weary tired. Sometimes optimism just took too much energy.

Tam, however, looked perkier, more alert, though her pain meds had her really groggy. I wondered how she could be so cheerful, so full of hope. Perhaps it was because her friends, some she hadn't seen in years, rallied around her and kept her involved with what was going on, with living. They left her no time for dying, not yet.

And though she insisted that Richard was only a very good friend, she couldn't help grinning at the mention of his name. I didn't know if their mutual attraction was going to be long-term or short-lived. I didn't care. So long as it made her happy, that was all that mattered.

As I waited for her to get the catheter implanted, I wanted to scream, "Hurry up! Get things moving. You've got to kill this thing before it kills her! It's growing and it's relentless."

The surgery to implant the catheter was uneventful. One end of the catheter went into her jugular vein, and the other end protruded from her upper middle chest. That end was divided into two ports, or lumens, so two different medications could be administered at different rates at the same time. The part that went into her jugular vein snaked around the base of her neck, just under her skin. It took me a while to get used to the sight of it—she looked so vulnerable. But it didn't seem to bother her at all.

When we got back to her house, Richard came loping across the street to see how she had come through the ordeal. Before I went home (Wayne and I lived an hour's drive away), Richard told me not to worry about Tam. He would keep an eye on her and let us know if she had any problems at all. He even brought over a big bowl of chicken soup for her to eat.

"It's very good for her, she has to keep her strength up," he said.

The time between her surgery on Friday and her first chemo session stretched over an eternity. My mood bounced up and down, from joy and relief that something was finally going to be done to despair that things were taking so long.

For this first chemo, she was hospitalized so the docs could see how well her body tolerated the drugs. She was supposed to get the Adriamycin and the ifosfamide for four days, then stay one more day to get the mesna.

One of the websites Tam found when she researched her possible treatment options said that a chemotherapy regimen usually includes drugs to fight cancer as well as drugs to help the patient cope with the side effects of the cancer-fighting drugs. Thus the Adriamycin and the ifosfamide were to kill the cancer cells, and the mesna was to help negate their side effects.

The oncology ward was very quiet, and the rooms were all private. Hers had a large window that gave her a clear view of the city and the mesa that stretched to the west beyond Albuquerque. Her room was equipped with a recliner as well as a bed and a TV with a VCR, and she had access to the patient lounge and a refrigerator well stocked with beverages and snacks. She said it was more like a vacation resort than a hospital.

And one of her buddies, Dick Fate, was in the room next door. Though his was a different kind of cancer from Tam's, it originated in just about the same place as Tam's, and he too had been very athletic. They were both Dr. Tarnower's patients; she had introduced them so he could offer Tammy encouragement and support. He had overcome his first bout with cancer a couple of years before Tammy had hers, and he had reassured her and helped her keep exercising so she could regain full use of her leg. His cancer too came back, this time just a month or so before Tammy's did. He was getting the same drugs as Tammy, only he had started on them several weeks before. He was completely bald—even his eyebrows and the hair on his arms were gone.

He was deeply depressed by the return of his cancer. He and his wife had two small children, and he worried about their future if he couldn't take care of them. Tammy was depressed about the return of her cancer too. But when the two of them got together in the hospital, they began to see the dark humor in their situations. They made morbid jokes and regaled the hospital staff with good-natured teasing. Dick Fate wore a silly Viking hat, complete with horns, on his bald head. Terri and her friend Mark brought Tammy a fake coonskin cap to wear.

"It isn't roadkill, either," Terri said. "No critter had to give its life for you. It's fake fur." And Tammy wore it, though she hadn't yet lost her hair.

The high point of their adventures was when they went bicycle riding in the hospital. One of Terri's coworkers, a friend to both Terri and Tammy, was an exercise physiologist named Kelvin Schenk. He came to visit and took Dick Fate and Tam, still hooked up to their IV poles, to the hospital's exercise room so they could go for a spin on the stationary bikes. I couldn't imagine either one of them having the energy, but Tammy said later that it made her feel so much better. She and Dick Fate both thought they were really tough, riding bikes in the hospital, even if it was only for a little while and the bikes didn't go anywhere.

After Tammy finished her first chemo session and got to go home, she began feeling better right away. For the first time in six weeks, she was able to drive a car. Ah, life was good again. And miracle of miracles, her HMO approved a referral for her to get radiation treatment at the Midwest Institute for Neutron Therapy at Fermilab (NTF) in Illinois.

According to Fermi's NTF website, neutron radiation has a 53 percent success rate against angiosarcoma tumors compared to a 38 percent success rate with conventional radiation. The difference was significant enough for her HMO to agree to refer her there.

I guess I was still operating in the numb mode. I was responding and reacting appropriately, but I had absolutely no initiative. I had no idea how to take control of the situation or even that such a thing was a possibility. I worried about finances but couldn't think of any way to come up with more money.

Terri, however, was able to think. She took over the decision making and said there were two things I needed to do. I needed to ask my uncle if he would loan me the money for Tam's trip to Illinois. And I needed to go with her. Nobody else in the family could do it. She and Cindy both had to work, or they would lose their jobs and their livelihoods. Wayne's health was too fragile for such a long trip. And Tammy certainly couldn't make the trip alone.

I readily agreed that she couldn't go alone. I had to think about it. I thought and pondered all night long, and by morning, I had the answers.

I asked Wayne if he would be okay if I went with Tam.

"Go!" he said. "You take care of Tam, and I'll take care of things here."

He would field phone calls and mail, keeping family and friends updated on what was going on with Tam and me. He would also keep the house in order and make sure the bills were paid on time.

As for how to pay for the trip, if I asked my uncle, who has more money than he or his progeny can spend in their lifetimes, I simply had to have a viable way to pay him back. And there was a way. Once my father's estate was settled, I could repay my uncle. Of course, it could take several years to sell property and settle the estate, but I was sure my uncle would accept the wait. I figured $20,000 would be enough to cover Tam's bills and pay for our trip to Illinois.

When I called my uncle and told him about Tam's situation, he immediately asked how much money we needed and when we needed it. The check came in the mail a couple of days later.

We were good to go. I shifted from being passive to being active, and it felt good. I knew what I had to do. I just had to fight a little to get it done.

Tam's hair started falling out about three weeks after her first chemo session—not just a hair here and there but in clumps. She knew it would happen, but when hair fell into her food, covered her pillow, and fogged into her eyes and mouth, she was appalled. She had it all shaved off to get this hair loss thing over with.

"I didn't expect it to be such a big deal," she said. "I know it sounds silly, but I feel kinda naked without it, more vulnerable, I guess. Now everybody can tell that I have cancer just by looking at me. I have no secrets anymore."

No wigs for Tammy, either. She opted for hats—tasteful hats, exotic hats, silly hats—as well as scarves and bandannas. Her friend Gretl Bernert had overcome breast cancer just the year before, and she gave Tam a large box of hats and scarves. Kelvin Schenk, who had taken her bike riding in the hospital, gave her a biker's bandanna, complete with the sweatband inside. It had a blazing yellow sun printed on a midnight-blue background dotted with stars. That sun sat smack-dab in the middle of the front, so it sat in the middle of her forehead when she wore it, which she did often.

I think she truly loved all those hats and bandannas and scarves. She loved wearing them; she didn't seem to resent the fact that she had to wear them or show her bald head. She was amazed by the fact that so many people cared for her enough to get them for her, that there were so many people who loved her.

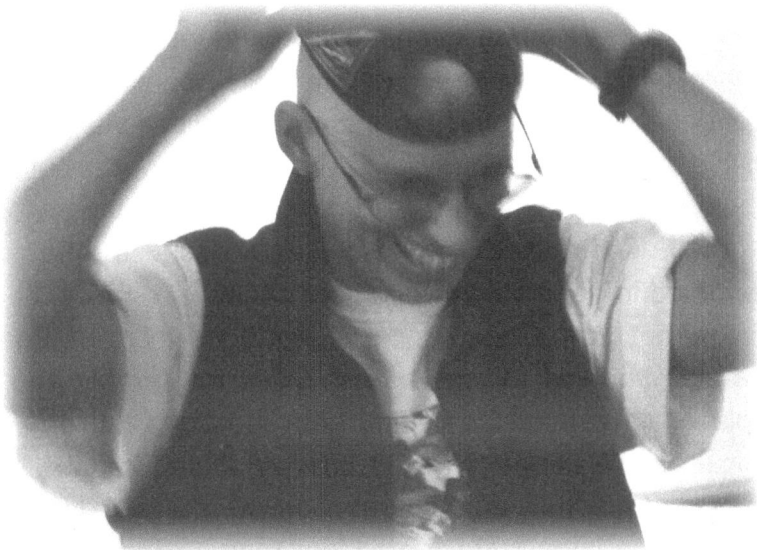

Tammy putting on her new biker's bandanna.

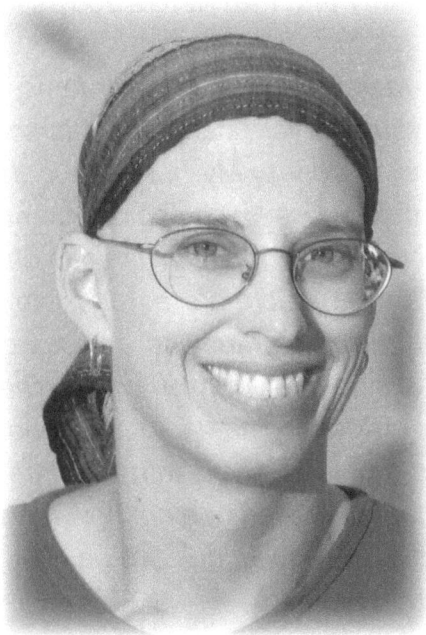

Bald Tammy wearing one of her favorite scarves.

"Hey, Mom, I found this website for people with cancer and their families," she said one day. "This website is devoted to cancer survivor stories, to show cancer patients that it's possible to beat this thing. Would you write a story about how we both survived the same weird cancer so we can post it?"

I think she asked me to write it because she was determined to get me involved in her cause.

When we posted our cancer story on the Internet, I gave my e-mail address to screen responses for Tammy and so people could contact us if they had questions, not to offer medical advice certainly but to offer encouragement. I was surprised at just how many responses we received. Usually I forwarded the ones that seemed legitimate to Tammy so she could respond too. Her information about cancer was much more current and accurate than mine.

A young woman named Jody sent an inquiry that deeply touched both Tammy and me. Here's Jody's first e-mail:

I hope this e-mail finds you and your family well. I just read the story about you and your daughter. It is so encouraging to read these types of stories. My husband is thirty-three years old and has been diagnosed with angiosarcoma. This is such a scary disease. Randy and I have only begun our journey in this. We are digging up as much info as possible. I have spoken with another lady whose father had angiosarcoma two years ago, and now she's been diagnosed with it. That's so scary . . . we have three children. The lady mentioned chromosome 26 being a gene that is involved with the hereditary aspect of sarcoma. She, her father, and one nephew have the gene.

Please let us know how things are going.

God bless and take care.

Jody

This is Tammy's e-mail response to Jody:

My mom forwarded me your e-mail. I think you are very wise to use all the resources available to you, including the Internet. I was also told that my tumor would most likely go to my lungs first, and my docs in Albuquerque were surprised to see it turn up in my tailbone. But when I went to a comprehensive cancer care center in Tucson, the oncologist there said they have seen several cases with angiosarcoma going to the spine. I think it's such a rare tumor that there really isn't enough known about it to pass judgment on where the stupid little beast can go or not.

It may sound kind of silly, but I really believe that a little hope goes a long way. From your e-mails it sounds like you're actively involved in Randy's care. I would like to encourage you to continue seeking out providers who have experience treating sarcomas. And in the meantime, love Randy as much as humanly possible and encourage his relatives and friends to do the same. Maybe with enough love, the beastly tumors will just have no reason to hang around.

Take care and keep in touch!

Tammy "Bald Is Beautiful" Redman

Falling hair wasn't the only side effect Tam endured with her chemotherapy. She developed persistent sores on the inside of her mouth, but Susan, her oncology nurse, was ready with medications to soothe them. And Tammy's ordinarily well-behaved intestines became clogged as though with cement. Again, more meds. Then the problem reversed, with no food lingering long enough for nutrients to be extracted before it was violently discharged. Finding a balance somewhere between constipation and diarrhea became an ongoing challenge. I think that was a turning point for Tammy, and she began to seek and use alternative natural remedies whenever possible to relieve her minor ills. They worked, and the side effects, if there were any, were much more tolerable for her.

We were able to catch up on Tammy's outstanding bills with the money from my uncle, but soon it looked as if it would have to be a choice between keeping up with all her bills or going to the Chicago area (to Batavia, Illinois, specifically) for neutron radiation. We had to do something about some of her bills.

The day came when Tammy could no longer afford to help make the house payment, and without her help, Terri couldn't afford the house. Reluctantly, Terri decided to put her house up for sale.

Tammy was horrified! She loved that house. She all but refused to consider moving. The relationship between Terri and Tammy rapidly degenerated until they were arguing most of the time.

Terri and one of her cycling buddies, Mark Mico, had become very good friends. He coached the high school cycling team as well as people who were serious triathlon contenders. It seemed he was as addicted to individual competitive sports and fitness as Terri was. On the Ts' birthday, Terri and Mark announced that they were going to be married. They spent more and more time together, and when they were at the house, Tam grumped at them both.

"Turn that thing down! I can't hear myself think," she yelled when they played CDs or watched television.

Tammy realized that she was depressed and that she was responsible for possibly more than her share of the problems she and Terri were having. She began counseling with Dr. Lewis Nemis, the psychologist she had seen on and off during her first bout with cancer.

After her first appointment with him this time, she told me that he had asked her if she was angry with Terri for being healthy, since they were twins and had always gone through more or less the same triumphs and ills until now.

"I don't think of myself as sick," she answered. "Sure, I have some serious problems right now, but that doesn't mean I'm really sick." Oh.

Nevertheless, I think he hit on a major cause of Tammy's problems with Terri. Besides, it looked like their comfortable situation was going to change with Terri's plans to marry. And as a result of Tammy's illness, the house she loved was going to be sold. So many things were changing, and Tammy had no control over them. She was angry, and as her twin and the person closest to her, Terri took the brunt of her anger.

In response, Terri became angry too and felt guilty. She spent more and more time away from home and felt guilty. Tam felt abandoned and angry. It became an almost hopeless, endless cycle, almost worse than the cancer.

Though Tammy knew Mark well, Wayne and I had never met him. One night, we arranged to meet him over dinner at a restaurant. Tammy came with us, and we arrived first. Soon Terri and Mark came striding up the walk, both wearing white shirts and jeans, both about the same height, and both laughing. He was a blond, blue-eyed Italian, his hair a sharp contrast to Terri's long dark-auburn hair. They didn't fawn all over each other, they didn't even touch, but it was obvious that there was a bond between them.

Mark was easygoing and easy to like, even though I came with hearty skepticism. With his joking and his obvious devotion for Terri, he won us over early on. We decided Terri could keep him, as if she really needed our approval.

The food was delicious, and everyone was in a jolly mood. We sat in a large booth, with Tam on one side of Mark and Terri on the other, and Wayne and I sitting opposite them.

Tam sat with her right elbow free, to Mark's right. He, like Terri, is left-handed. The three joked and teased and laughed. Wayne and I were included, but it was almost as though the three of them were tuned to the same private wavelength. It was like old times with Tam and Terri, and we all had a grand time.

Finances continued to devil Tammy. After consulting with a financial advisor, she decided to swallow her pride and file for bankruptcy. We would pay off her student loan with the money from my uncle, and somehow we would keep up with her car payments. But the credit card debt would go.

She had to appear before a bankruptcy judge. When her name was called, she stood and walked to the front of the room. As I watched her, tall and gaunt, her face gray and her bald head covered with a scarf, I cried. She looked so very sick, and she was. The judge simply asked her to verify her name, then granted the bankruptcy.

Tam's financial problems were supposed to be over then, but they weren't really. Although by law her creditors were supposed to leave her alone, they didn't. They called day and night, threatening her with all sorts of things. She knew they couldn't do anything but harass her, but it still made her feel ashamed. Terri fielded the calls when she was home, but she wasn't there much of the time.

Tam was cleared to seek treatment at the Fermi Neutron Therapy Facility in Illinois. It was closed for annual maintenance for most of the month of October, but Tam had an appointment with a radiation oncologist there on October 31.

She finally accepted the fact that the house had to be sold, and she wanted to be settled into her own apartment before we went to Chicago. She pored over the classified ads in the newspaper, made dozens of phone calls, and finally narrowed her search to a few places she thought she could afford. On a Saturday morning, Terri went with her to check them out. They found the perfect apartment, across the street from the Albuquerque Botanic Gardens and Aquarium and with a golf course as the backyard. It was on the third floor, and treetops framed views from the back windows. A small balcony overlooked the golf course. Clerestory windows in the living room made it bright and airy.

"Tam, this is perfect!'" Terri said. "You have to get this one. The rent may be a bit steep, but I can help pay it."

When I saw it, I could see why they fell in love with the place. But it was on the third floor! I reminded Tam that she had a few little problems with her back, and those two long flights of stairs might prove challenging. "I can still climb stairs," she said. "Besides, I won't be having back problems forever, and I feel safer up here, above the ground floor."

From Tammy's journal:

September 21, 2001

I found a cute little apartment that I'll be moving into for the next few weeks. The apartment is downtown, by the river and the botanical gardens. I'm kind of excited about it. I'll get the keys tomorrow, but I won't be staying there until after October 12. Then I'll be doing my fourth round of chemo on October 15. I think the month of October will go very fast.

###

Terri, Cindy, and Cindy's two daughters, Heather and Chelsea, helped Tam pack. We hired a local moving company to haul her stuff up those stairs, then her dad reassembled all the things that had been taken apart for the move and hung her bulletin board over her computer desk. I helped her unpack and get settled.

Cindy called the apartment Tammy's Tree House. Oscar, Tam's cat, loved watching birds flit through the branches of the trees outside the windows. And she could negotiate those stairs with no problem at all. I think I was the only one bothered by the stairs, but they were probably good for me.

On Tuesday, September 4, Tam started her second chemo session. She didn't have to be hospitalized for this one. She drove herself to the medical center, made her way up to the oncology/hematology department, and settled into one of the comfy recliners reserved for people getting chemotherapy. Susan, her oncology nurse, was a very tiny, wiry lady who had to crane her neck to peer up into Tammy's face unless Tam was sitting in a recliner—then they were nearly eye-to-eye.

That day there were four nurses working the oncology room, and the ambience in that room, because of those four, was surprisingly upbeat and cheerful. There was much laughter, some tears, and genuine concern for everyone, or so it seemed to me. There was very little of the we're-just-too-busy-to-bother-with-you attitude that Tam had been subjected to with some of her other medical encounters.

And everybody, whether patient or someone with the patient, was hugged when they came in and again when they left. I frankly thought it was carrying things a bit far at first, but I came to look forward to those hugs almost as much as Tammy did.

From Tammy's journal:

September 26, 2001

I'm doing pretty well, all things considered. Last week I had an MRI of my low spine and pelvis. The pelvis MRI showed that the beasties in my right SI joint and iliac crest are shrinking. Also, the tumors in my S1 and L5 vertebrae haven't gotten any bigger. This is after only two chemo cycles. This week, I'm in the middle of my third chemo cycle. I'm starting to feel a little tired but not too bad. There are so many things to help deal with the side effects—GCSF (Neupogen), some kind of red-cell growth factor (Procrit), blood transfusions, antinausea meds, and good old-fashioned saline. My nurse is so good about getting me whatever I need, even if I don't know what to ask for.

I'll get a fourth round of chemo in the middle of October. Then on October 30—I can't believe it—I get to go to the Fermilab for neutron therapy in Illinois. My mom and I will be there for about six weeks, and I'll be getting a total of twelve treatments. Neutron therapy is supposed to be particularly effective at zapping sarcomas. After that, I'm not too sure what will happen. I'll probably get two more chemo cycles and plastic surgery on my back. Then the tumor on my left leg will have to be dealt with.

So I've still got a long way to go. But I'm hopeful that I may have a chance at some kind of recovery since the chemo seems to be having an effect.

I don't remember who said it first—I think it was probably Wayne—but one day, Tam said she was hungry for a milk shake from the Dairy Queen, and he answered, "Whatever the hell you want, babe!" That became our unofficial motto. Tam never seemed to take unfair advantage of it. She tried to be very frugal with her requests. But she openly asked for any and all treatment options that might offer hope, and we all did our best to make them available to her, one way or another. There were little things like the leopard-print flannel pajamas from Penneys and the small square tiger-face pillow from Walgreens for her to put behind her back—things we got for her just because we thought she'd like them, and she loved them.

Richard visited her often in her new apartment. He brought her a small stereo CD player so they could listen to music. She loved music, all kinds of music. She and Terri had gone through the University of Hawaii on music scholarships. She had a collection of hundreds of CDs, and she and Richard spent hours listening to them and talking. He wasn't put off in the least by her bald head.

One weekend he went camping with his two kids. He invited Tam to come along, but she didn't have the energy to go, although she certainly wanted to go. She was a bit depressed by the whole situation.

That Sunday, Cindy and I took her to the movies. Tam wanted to see *The Others,* with Nicole Kidman, so that's what we saw. Poor choice! It was a good movie but very dark and very depressing.

After the movie, Tammy was in a foul mood. She grumped about the tiniest details, about things that mattered not at all. Until then, she had been so very good. She had taken this whole cancer thing much better than the rest of us, refusing to let it get her down, at least most of the time. She had been sad sometimes and scared, but she had never been, well, mean (except to Terri).

But that weekend, she made up for lost time. She had asked for some grapes from the grapevines in our backyard, then she got angry because I brought too many. She yelled at Cindy for taking too long to get iced tea from the refrigerator. And she was positively livid at the mere sight of Terri. She was so very over the top that we couldn't help grinning as we dodged her wrath.

On Monday, Richard returned, and her mood mellowed. By Tuesday, she conceded that she had perhaps been a little grumpy.

-6-

The closer it got to October 30, our departure date, the crazier things got.

On Monday, October 15, one end of Tam's catheter was somehow pulled out in the night. The hole it left behind didn't bleed much, and she was too groggy to worry about it till morning.

Dr. Tarnower was appalled that Tam had waited so long to call her!

"That is the kind of thing you go to the emergency room to get taken care of immediately. You could have bled to death before morning!" she scolded. I drove Tammy to the hospital to have another catheter implanted.

On Friday, October 26, just four days before we were scheduled to leave for Chicago, Tammy woke up with a sore throat.

"Mom, it hurts from my lips to my butt!" she said when she called that morning. Then she called the doctor, who ordered industrial-strength antibiotics for her.

They did the job, and we took off for Chicago as planned. We were both so excited we were almost giddy. We were off to a new and strange part of the country we had never seen before. Tam had found us very cheap plane tickets on the Internet—both our round-trip tickets cost less than a one-way ticket for just one of us from an airline ticket office. Best of all, we just knew, really knew, that neutron therapy would do the trick and kill Tam's cancer. We just knew she would walk away as good as new, or nearly so.

It had been only a month and a half since the infamous events of 9/11, and airport security was intense. We both had to take off our shoes for inspection. Tam's spine was so stiff she could no longer bend down to take hers off or put them on without sitting down, so I did it for her. That aroused suspicion. She was given a thorough personal examination. The fact that she was totally bald and obviously sick made no impression on them at all; they seemed to think it was a ploy to distract them, that it was something sinister. Our carry-ons were opened, and everything was left in shambles. We had to repack before we could proceed to the plane, but we made our flight with minutes to spare.

When we landed in Chicago, we rented a car for a month, then made our way to our hotel in Naperville. I did the driving, and Tam navigated with the use of the simple map the car rental agency had given us. The car was a tiny, gutless compact with rather timid brakes, but we were so happy to be there we didn't care.

Our room was equipped with a small kitchenette, so we quickly unpacked and went in search of a grocery store. Once we found one, we bought enough staples, things like cereal, tea (for both of us), and coffee (just for me—Tam didn't touch the stuff) and canned things to last us the month we planned to stay.

Driving was different in the Chicago area than it was at home in New Mexico, and it took us a while to adapt to those differences. We were barreling along what looked like a freeway when suddenly traffic slowed, and we were accosted by a tollbooth. *Oh damn, what do we do now?* I wondered. Tam read the signs as I panicked and looked to see what other drivers were doing. Actually, there were many tollbooths stretching across the roadway, one for each lane of traffic. Fortunately, this one was manned—or rather, womanned—and Tam dug a dollar bill out of her wallet, and I handed it to the toll taker. She seemed satisfied and handed me change.

We had gone only a few miles when we came upon another tollbooth, only there was no one in sight at this one. There was only a metal scoop protruding into my traffic lane—they actually expected me to toss coins into the damned thing! I tried and missed. The ground around the thing was littered with coins, not all of them ours. Tam dug for more coins, and I got out and put them in this time, as traffic behind us backed up and horns honked. Finally the gate lifted, and we drove on.

Chicago traffic <u>moved</u>! I'm not sure what would have happened to us if we hadn't kept up. I was afraid to find out. At home I have a reputation as the Lead Foot Queen of the civilized world, but these people drove so fast they scared even me. And they used their horns—a lot. But they actually backed off to let me change lanes or meld into traffic from an on-ramp. And they didn't tailgate. Once I got used to the speed and the tollgates, circulation returned in my knuckles, and I noticed that drivers there were actually quite courteous, so long as I didn't slow down.

By some miracle, we arrived at the Fermilab in Batavia and made our way to the Neutron Therapy Facility on time. It wasn't at all what I expected. There was a long reflection pond dotted with wild ducks and geese in front of a very tall, tapered building with two tall arms that converged at the top. Flags from various countries were flying in a row along the front. We followed the signs and drove around to the back of the main building and down another long drive flanked with squat cement buildings. Finally, we came to the one that had a small sign on the front that read Neutron Therapy. This place was designed as a working physics laboratory; patient treatment was apparently an afterthought or a sideline.

Finding the building was relatively easy. Finding the door wasn't. It was tucked behind a cement panel that arched to the top of the building. I suppose that kept the snow from piling up outside the door, as well as softened the look of an otherwise utilitarian cement box of a building. Once inside, we made our way down a walkway with large, menacing clanking machines on either side. I was afraid that if I ventured from the cement walkway, unknown disaster would result—one of the machines might devour us.

We finally found a door with a sign that read Neutron Therapy. Through the door there was a very nice waiting room, though it was fairly small. The blue upholstered chairs were comfortable, but there were only ten or so of them in the long, narrow room. One wall was glass, and it looked out onto a small courtyard with shrubs still green in the late October sun. Birds bustled around the feeders placed among the bushes. A coffee machine sat on a table at one end of the room, and a short, no-nonsense receptionist worked at her desk at the other end.

I was thoroughly intimidated by this whole place, ready to turn around and run away. Tammy, however, wasn't. She checked in, completed the paperwork, and answered questions as though none of this was at all out of the ordinary.

At about 8:30 a.m., she was called in to talk to Dr. Jeffrey Shafer, a radiation oncologist. I was invited to go with her if I wished, and of course I did.

Dr. Shafer was a tall, lean man in his midfifties. His dark hair was tinged with gray, and it stuck out here and there where it refused to be tamed by his morning grooming efforts.

His sharply pressed khakis were a bit frayed at the bottom, and he wore a red-and-black Mickey Mouse tie. Obviously he was a very easygoing man, no ego problems here.

For well over an hour, he pushed for all the details, both monumental and minute, of Tam's cancer evolution. He wasn't rushed or distracted; he was completely focused on Tam and what she had to say. After only a few minutes of watching and listening to him, I felt sure that if anybody could help her beat this thing, this man could.

"The chemo and the radiation together may be a problem," he said. "The most powerful beam in the world is here, at Fermi. It's tough, neutrons and Adriamycin. You can finish the chemo first, or we can sandwich radiation between chemo treatments. We want to exploit what works, get the most mileage out of treatment with the least cost, in terms of side effects to you.

"I've been in oncology for twenty-seven years. You learn to observe little things, you develop an intuition. Hang with me."

After spending an hour or so with us, he left to place a call to Tam's oncologist in Albuquerque. About twenty minutes later, he came back in the room to give us his conclusions: Tammy's cancer was not local—it was systemic. And it was pervasive. There were three, possibly four, areas of tumor. There was probably no area of overlap with her previous radiation, which was a great plus.

He said that the key to treatment is providing local/regional control with radiation and systemic treatment with chemotherapy.

"Your pain distresses me a little bit," Shafer said.

"I don't know if the pain is caused by the tumor or by the changes in the tumor caused by the chemo," Tammy responded.

"It could be caused by the bones crumbling," he said. Oh.

He wanted to see the films of her first radiation so he could avoid any overlap with the neutron radiation treatment. There could be no overlap because that would kill all the tissue and bone in its path.

Tammy had been thrown into early menopause after her first series of radiation treatments, but when she talked to the radiation oncologist who administered them, he said that the radiation couldn't possibly have caused it. So Tam asked Shafer if the earlier radiation could have caused her ovaries to shut down.

Dr. Shafer said, "We're gonna find out, but it certainly could have been the radiation."

Tammy's suspicions were confirmed. "You know, I might not have had kids anyway, but I would have liked to have had a choice," she said to me later on the way home.

"Angios are crazy, an MRI can be wrong," Shafer continued. "We try to make treatment areas very specific. Neutrons focus on known tumor. We need to identify that specifically. We need the best imaging possible. We'll do a PET scan, including your lungs and liver. We want to include everything that lights up in our treatment."

He wanted us to get the PET (positron emission tomography) scan in Chicago before she started treatment.

"Chicago is a great place to see," he said. "This is the premier high-energy physics lab in the world, soon to be outdone by a facility in Lucerne, Switzerland. We have the only upright scanner in the world. It scans the patient while the patient is standing." Because the patient had to be standing, or at least propped up during neutron radiation therapy, this allowed physicians and technicians to see exactly what would be exposed to the radiation and how to adjust impact angles to most effectively nuke the tumors.

Tam had the upright scan right after her visit with Dr. Shafer so he could work on designing her treatment plan.

Just the facts, no histrionics, no pity, no hand-wringing. Just the facts, no patronizing or talking down to us. But no proclamations of doom either. Hope, always hope.

This was not a defeat—it was a challenge.

But we went home to Albuquerque without her receiving treatment—not yet. After going over her records in detail and after talking with Dr. Tarnower on the phone, Dr. Shafer decided to send Tam home for two or three more chemo sessions before she started neutron therapy.

I wanted to shout, "But that's why we're here! It took so much for us to get here. We have all these reservations and we're going home empty-handed?" But I said nothing. This was the best course of action for Tam, and that was what the whole thing was about, after all.

Shafer said that since the chemo seemed to be working, it would be folly to stop before it was finished. We were to come back after the chemo regimen was over. She would have a PET scan and start treatment right away. "We'll nuke everything that glows," he said, "including any tumors that may not have been found before."

I worried about coping with the snow and ice of a Chicago winter, but there was simply no choice if Tam was going to survive.

We went back to our hotel and told them that we wouldn't be staying a month, after all. We were going back home the next day. Then we went to our room and took our food stash out of the cupboards and stacked it on the counter for the hotel staff. We decided to leave the perishables in the refrigerator. Surely someone at the hotel would be able to use it—we certainly couldn't take all that with us on the plane.

It wasn't easy getting our plane reservations changed. Since we had discount tickets, we couldn't change our return tickets or have them refunded. When I explained that we hadn't planned to cut our stay short but that it was medically necessary, the people at the airline were unimpressed. They said that Tam's cancer was a preexisting condition, after all. We should have realized this was a possibility. They were not responsible, and they would not allow us to use our return ticket early. With help from the people at Fermi, we finally got return tickets on Southwest Airlines. They gave us a deep discount despite the short notice. Their seats were roomier than those on our flight to Chicago too and much more comfortable for Tam and her long, long legs.

We returned home on November 1. Wayne and I celebrated our forty-fourth wedding anniversary together, after all.

The months of November and December were spent in limbo—for me, anyway—and, I suspect, for Tammy too. No matter where I was or what I was doing, I felt as though I should be somewhere else doing something different. We went to movies, we visited with friends, we went about the ordinary business of day-to-day life, but I felt detached. I felt that I really should have been in Chicago getting Tammy's cancer knocked out once and for all.

Richard visited Tammy at her "tree house" apartment often. They sat in her living room and watched winter come to the tall trees outside her third-story window, and they talked. He brought her concoctions of vegetable and fruit juices to boost her immune system. He brought her happiness.

Terri spent hours with her up in that apartment too, just talking or doing the chores that were becoming more difficult for Tammy to do for herself as her spine became stiffer. She carried trash down to the Dumpster. She cleaned the bathroom and changed the cats' litter boxes. (Tam took Terri's two cats to live with her and her cat, Oscar, soon after she moved to her apartment.)

Tammy couldn't lift even moderately heavy things anymore, so Terri took her grocery shopping, then carried the groceries upstairs and put them away for her. Though lifting and deep bending were feats she could no longer accomplish with her fragile, stiff spine, getting up and down those stairs was never a problem for her. I think she actually enjoyed it; it was one form of exercise she could still do.

The day after Thanksgiving, Cindy treated the girls in the family to a live performance of The Nutcracker Suite. The ballet was delightful, the mood was festive, and Tammy had a grand time, as did we all.

From Tammy's journal:

November 26, 2001

Here's what's been going on: I went to Chicago at the beginning of the month and talked with a radiation oncologist. He was very encouraging, but he thought my prognosis would be best if I went back to Albuquerque and finished all my chemo treatments before getting radiation. I was pretty bummed because it was tricky getting the health insurance referral and the cash together to come for the consultation. I didn't know if I could do it again. So I came back to Albuquerque, and three weeks ago, I had my fifth chemo. I was getting really hammered. I got a blood transfusion and felt much better. My sixth chemo was supposed to be Monday, but my doc said it might be a good idea to wait a week so I'll be feeling better. So I get the sixth chemo next Monday (December 3). I plan on really enjoying this week.

###

Tam's insurance company insisted that she have the PET scan done in Albuquerque rather than in Chicago. There was only one machine available through her HMO; it was at the Veterans Administration Hospital. She had to scramble to get it done before we left for Chicago again.

We were ecstatic with the results. The scan showed that all her tumors were dead. Both Tarnower and Shafer, however, wanted Tammy to have the neutron radiation anyway to kill any errant cancer cells that may be lurking in the shadows somewhere.

We planned to leave for Chicago on January 7 and return on February 7. But this time, we paid a bit more for our tickets so we could change them if we needed to without the hassle we had last time.

-7-

January 7 came at last, and at 9:35 a.m., we boarded a plane bound for Chicago. This time, we knew what to expect from all the security procedures, and we arrived at the airport early enough to accommodate them. This time, we rented a midsize car, a Chevrolet Impala. It had plenty of room for Tammy's long legs, enough acceleration to get out of the way in traffic, and brakes that actually stopped the car when I stepped on the brake pedal.

The same hotel we had stayed in the first time welcomed us back with a room on the third floor. The hotel was in Naperville but near the highway, so it took only about fifteen minutes to get to Fermilab in Batavia, a town located forty miles west of Chicago.

Tammy's appointment at Fermi was at 2:00 p.m. the next day, a Tuesday. We assumed that we would see Dr. Shafer again, but we didn't. We saw a Dr. Smoron this time. He was very nice, but he wasn't at all familiar with Tam's case and was unprepared to answer her questions. I had the feeling that he was verbally patting us on the head until Dr. Shafer was available, and that would not be until Friday. The good news was that Shafer had finished calculating Tam's treatment plan. She would be able to start treatment right after she saw him on Friday. We had hoped to get started Tuesday, but Friday was better than not having treatment at all.

We left Fermi that afternoon a bit disappointed but still excited to be there again. We headed for the grocery store to lay in supplies, but not so many this time—just enough to get us through a couple of days. I was driving with enough confidence to almost feel comfortable as I tried to keep up with traffic.

I was sure I knew just how to find the grocery store again. After all, it was only a mile or so from our hotel. I got off at the exit near our hotel and drove—and drove and drove. We were amazed at how there could be so many people living there and still have so much forested land left so near metropolitan Chicago. We drove through little villages and over streams and on and on. Finally I glanced down at the odometer. We had driven fifty miles since I turned off the highway.

I had turned the wrong way.

"Mom, you know what your problem is?" Tammy said. "You have no sense of 'where'—where things are, where to go to get there. But that's okay, that's why God invented maps. We'll get there."

And we did. The first thing we bought was a detailed map of the area, as well as another plastic-laminated map that showed the main thoroughfares. Before that, Tammy had insisted on sharing the driving chores with me for short trips—just to prove to herself she could still do it, I suspect. After that, she never again got in the driver's seat. I assumed that was because it was too hard for her to push the brake pedal any more, but in retrospect, it was probably also because she didn't trust my navigation skills. I could get the car down the road okay, but I don't think she trusted me to read the map. That probably saved us a lot of unnecessary confusion.

When we paid for our groceries, we got an extra $5 worth of change—quarters mostly but also dimes and nickels. The car's ashtray was clean, so that's where we put our change stash. Now we were ready for those tollbooths. We were careful to put all spare change in the ashtray so we wouldn't again be caught unprepared. Perhaps now it wouldn't be so obvious that we were outlanders.

The next day, since we had nothing scheduled, we decided to be tourists and look around. First we wanted to check out the Fermilab to see what else it had to offer, particularly that fascinating tall building at the entrance. I was concerned that we would wander onto a restricted area and get into serious trouble. After all, we had to check in and get badges just to get onto the site and go to the Neutron Therapy Facility.

"They'll let us know if we go onto a restricted area," Tammy assured me.

We started with the large, squat building where we had checked in. We found out that it was the Lederman Education Center, which explained the school buses in the parking lot. Inside, besides the reception desk, there were exhibits, a small gift shop area, and a long hallway lined with doors that led into other rooms, probably where the kids went to learn about this place and about science, particularly about physics.

We picked up several brochures that explained just what Fermilab was all about, then went on to Wilson Hall. Wilson Hall and the Lederman Center were the only two buildings in the entire complex that were open to the public.

Fermilab

Wilson Hall was sixteen stories high, and the two converging wings of the building were separated by an atrium that extended up in the center of the structure. Crossovers connected the two towers on some of the floors. Besides the information desk in the atrium, there were offices and a cafeteria and a giant pendulum called the Foucault pendulum, suspended on a fifty-two-meter cable from the top of the atrium. The earth's rotation and gravity kept it slowly swinging back and forth, so the little placard said. We just stood there and watched it swing, awed that such a thing was possible. It was probably the closest thing to perpetual motion we would ever see.

And of course, there were full-sized trees and plants growing as if they were at home in their native jungle; it even smelled like a jungle, earthy and green.

A wide staircase led from the first floor to the second, where there was an art gallery. Though windows from the rooms on all floors opened onto the atrium, most floors were off-limits to the public. Wilson Hall was the central laboratory building and a place for visiting scientists to gather. We were welcome, however, to take the elevator to the fifteenth-floor observation deck. Part of it was under construction, but we could still look out over much of the six-thousand-eight-hundred-acre site.

These people were proud of their work with high-energy physics, and they seemed determined to help us understand just what that was. Exhibits mounted near each window explained what we were looking at outside. There were even models showing the various buildings and structures. An Internet kiosk gave visitors access to yet more information. Tantalizing information, but always there were the secret things, the questions we could not ask, the places we could not see, hints of darker things lurking in the background.

They used words like *quark* and *proton* and *neutrino* and *dark matter*. I was impressed, but I had no idea what they were talking about. I was getting tired. I'm sure Tammy was too, but she wanted to read every word on every display before we left.

A brochure about the history of the place said that in 1966, the town of Weston, Illinois, was selected as the site of a new National Accelerator Laboratory. The Universities Research Association was formed to run the new laboratory for the US

Department of Energy. The URA is a corporation of eighty-nine universities in the United States, Canada, Japan, and Italy.

The primary mission of the National Accelerator Laboratory, now known as Fermilab, is to "advance the understanding of the fundamental nature of matter and energy," according to one booklet we found there. The motto on a general map of the place reads, "Discovering the nature of nature." Okay, that much I could understand.

Construction of the linear accelerator (linac) began in 1968. In 1974, the laboratory was renamed the Fermi National Accelerator Laboratory, or the Fermilab, in honor of Italian physicist Enrico Fermi, who won the Nobel Prize for Physics in 1938. He was a major player in the development of atomic energy. According to one of the booklets, "in the squash courts under the west stand of the University of Chicago's Stagg Field, Fermi supervised the design and assembly of an 'atomic pile,' a code word for an assembly that in peacetime would be known as a nuclear reactor."

Early on, it became obvious that the linac could "accelerate and deliver" more beam than was necessary to support the high-energy physics program, and Fermi scientists wondered if some of it could be diverted for medical use. The protons could be used to produce neutrons to treat cancers that didn't respond to conventional photon or X-ray radiation. The National Cancer Institute funded clinical trials at Fermi from 1976 to 1985.

One of the medical researchers in the project, Dr. Frank Henderson, described the difference between the two types of radiation this way:

"The effect of photons is like one thousand ping-pong balls entering a room and bouncing around. Now put the same amount of energy into one bowling ball. That's the neutrons. If they strike a part of the DNA, it cannot be repaired by the cells. The damage done by photons can often be repaired."

We had come to the right place to kill off Tammy's cancer.

One of the most prominent views from the observation deck was a ring of water four miles across. The water covered the Tevatron, a superconducting accelerator that was transformed into a proton-antiproton collider. The Tevatron was buried twenty feet below the surface and was topped with the ring of water. That water was evidently warmer than other ponds and lakes nearby because they sometimes iced over, but that ring of water never did. Consequently, it was nearly always covered with flocks of wild ducks and geese.

From the fifteenth-floor windows, we could see small lakes and stands of trees. We could also see what looked like a herd of buffalo off in the distance. And that is exactly what it was. According to the text on one exhibit, over one thousand acres of the site are dedicated to restoring the tall grass prairie that was native to the area before so many humans and so many of their structures destroyed it. The buffalo were a part of that effort. A small herd of fifty or so of the beasts roamed over a ninety-acre portion of the site.

The more we learned about the Fermilab, the more paradoxical it seemed. The people there were working on top-secret projects, yet they eagerly shared much of their knowledge with the public. Access to parts of the six-thousand-eight-hundred-acre site was strictly off-limits, but much of the land was designed to attract public use. There were bike trails and hiking trails everywhere, and the lakes were open to canoeing when the weather allowed. On weekends, there were nature programs for the general public. With the exception of Wilson Hall, all the structures were no-nonsense utilitarian, yet huge pieces of free-form sculptures dotted the site. It seemed dedicated to promoting the study and sheer joy of science, with a little art thrown in for good measure.

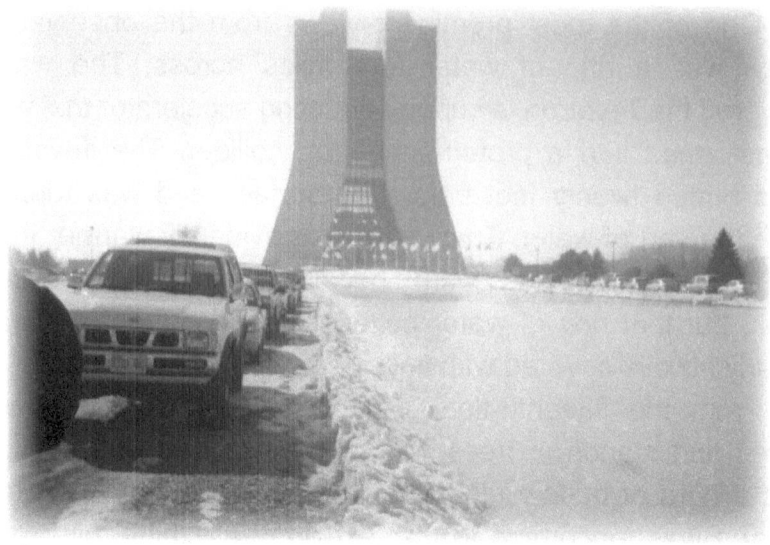

Wilson Hall and snow at Fermilab.

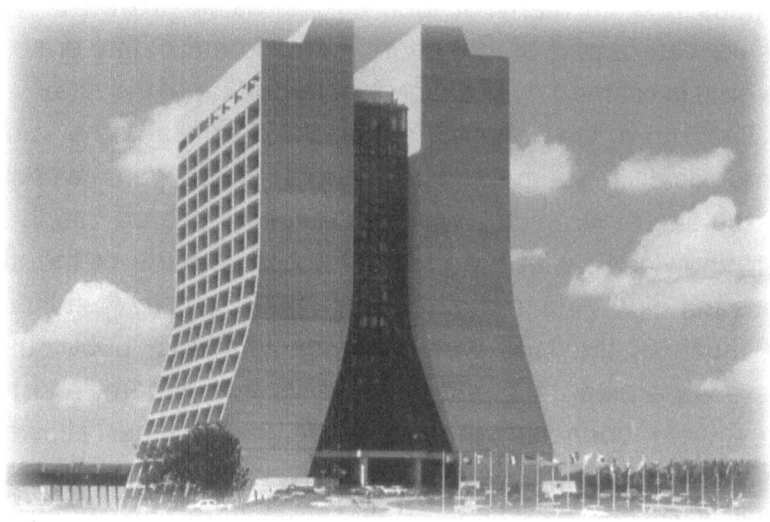

Wilson Hall in the summer. (This is a postcard photo.)

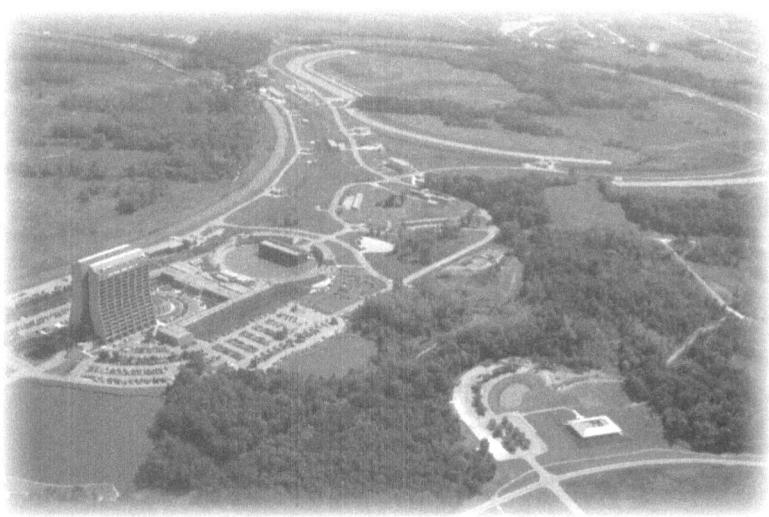

An aerial view of part of the Fermilab's 6800 acres, including
Wilson hall. (Photo from a postcard.)

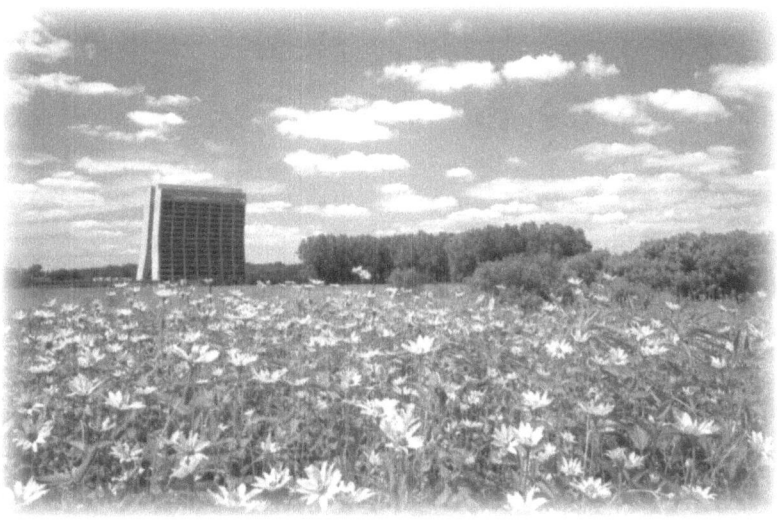

Another view of Wilson Hall. (Photo from a postcard.)

Finally, Tammy's curiosity was satisfied for the day, and we went back to our hotel room. But that wasn't our last visit to the observation deck—we came back several times while Tammy was undergoing treatment, and each time, we learned things we had overlooked earlier.

Since Tam had treatments only three times a week, that left plenty of time for us to explore and enjoy being tourists. We had been urged by the people at the hotel to take the commuter train downtown. Traffic was atrocious, they said, and finding a parking space was nearly impossible. But we were both concerned about Tammy's spine getting damaged even further by the jostling crowds on the train, so we opted to drive anyway. With Tammy navigating and me determined not to be intimidated by the traffic or by Tammy, we made it.

We visited the Shedd Aquarium, and we walked along the shores of Lake Michigan. We had been warned that the lakeshore was bitter cold in the wintertime, but that day, the weather was still relatively mild, and our walk along the shore was delightful. It was the first time I had seen a lake so large that you couldn't see the opposite shore. It looked just like the ocean, with waves lapping at the sandy beach. It even sounded like the ocean. The only thing missing was the salty smell in the air. There were just a half dozen or so other people on the beach. The sun was shining, and the breeze was gentle. Surely this was a portent of good things to come.

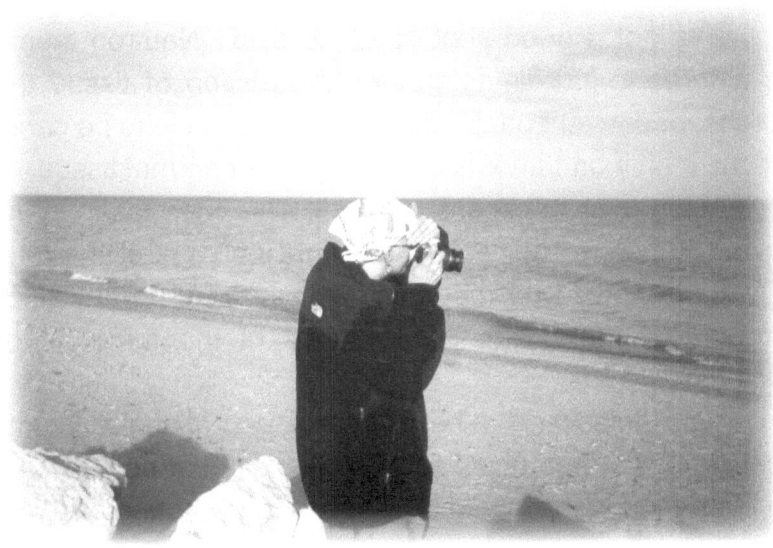

Lake Michigan. Tam loved taking photos of the lake.

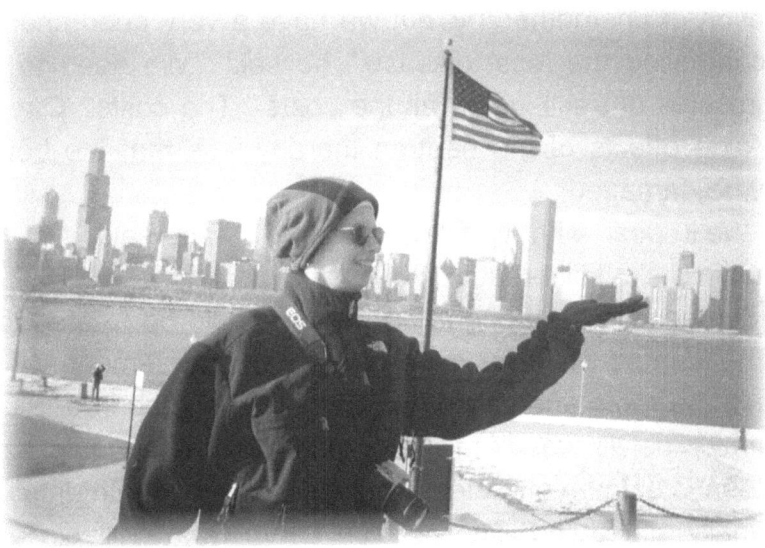

Tammy enjoying the sights in Chicago.

Friday afternoon, January 11, Tammy was finally able to see Dr. Shafer again.

"We've got a good shot at it," he said. "Neutron therapy has a three-to-four-times-greater destruction of tissue than photons, or conventional radiation. We just have to be careful to focus it only on tumor tissue and protect normal tissue."

He went over the scans with her. The ones taken in July showed tumors in her spine and right pelvis. But the latest PET scan showed no metabolic activity at all in any of the tumors, and there was no evidence of the tumor in her pelvis.

He said, however, that he was suspicious of angiosarcomas because they are so unpredictable. He said that he was afraid that even though they were shut down, the tumors might come back. So he wanted to nuke all tumor sites, even the one in her pelvis.

"You have metastatic disease. System control is a function of chemotherapy, but we have a very good chance of controlling the local disease," he said. "We need to be aggressive but still weigh all the costs." The costs? One of the side effects of the neutron therapy was that the bowel may be damaged.

"We'll deal with it if we have to," Tam said. "In the meantime, I'm still breathing!"

Shafer said he thought the pelvis should be treated too, but he wanted Dr. Tarnower's opinion and agreement. When he left the room and called her, he got it—she agreed. Since Tammy's pelvis wasn't in the original plan, she would have thirteen treatments instead of the twelve treatments as originally scheduled. The neutron beam was available only three days a week, so that meant we would have to stay a few extra days. Thank goodness we had flexible airline reservations this time.

"I'd like you to be on vitamin E, one thousand milligrams, it's an antioxidant," Shafer said, "and selenium and green tea, lots of green tea. Whatever you're doing, you're doing something right. It looks great."

When I asked him about stabilizing Tammy's back after the radiation for the trip home, Shafer said he didn't think she would need it. Nor did he think she would need surgery to stabilize her spine later.

"Give it three months to fill in after treatment," he said. "Bony tissue should fill in without any further treatment. For now, though, don't fall!"

Then Tammy changed into a hospital gown and prepared for her first neutron radiation session.

The treatment room was a surprise, yet another example of the no-frills, nothing-wasted attitude at this place. It was a converted freight elevator that had once been used to lower equipment into the accelerator tunnel. Now the elevator / treatment room was used to lower patients down into the neutron beam line. Long concrete cones were used to shape the beam to the patient's anatomy and limit exposure to healthy tissue.

To create the neutron beam, two magnets divert a fraction of the linac proton beam, bend it around a ninety-degree curve, and direct it toward a beryllium target outside the freight elevator, producing what they call fast neutrons. The resulting neutron beam is manipulated and sharply focused to target only the tumor area, not surrounding healthy tissue.

I waited by the coffee pot, pretending to read, while Tammy had her first treatment. She was gone for what seemed like forever, nearly an hour.

When she finally reappeared, she grinned and said, "Am I glowing yet?"

She had a totally militant attitude about this cancer. She considered any peripheral damage that might be incurred by treatment a necessary cost of the war she was waging. The monumental power of neutrons and the equipment that delivered them elicited only curiosity, no trepidation whatsoever. Cancer was her enemy, and she was determined to vanquish it, no matter the cost.

That night we ate at a restaurant in the nearby strip center to celebrate. The neutron beam was only available on Tuesdays, Wednesdays and Fridays, so we had the next three days to explore.

Chicago

Saturday morning, we once again braved Chicago traffic and went to see the Chicago Institute of Art. It was magnificent! And huge—there was so much to see. We tried to see it all, but we didn't have enough time or energy. The museum was hosting an exhibit entitled Van Gogh and Gauguin, the Studio of the South, so we got in line to see it. We waited half an hour or so as the line inched forward. When we finally reached the doorway, we discovered that we needed special tickets to enter. So we returned to the ticket counter at the entrance to the museum and got in another line to purchase the tickets. Alas, when we finally got to the front of that line, we didn't have enough cash with us to buy the tickets. I hadn't brought credit cards—I had left them at the hotel so we wouldn't be totally stranded if I should lose my wallet.

We gave up on the Van Gogh and Gauguin exhibit; there was more to see than we had time for anyway. But we did pick up brochures about it so we could see what we'd missed when we got back to our room. That night we ate macaroni and cheese and applesauce for dinner, comfort food for our wounded egos. I felt like a true country bumpkin after the Van Gogh-Gauguin fiasco.

Next we took in the Field Museum, another wondrous place. It had everything, from miniature dollhouses to dinosaurs. Tammy spent hours perusing an exhibit of ancient Egyptian artifacts, but her very favorite exhibit was Sue, billed as "the world's largest, most complete, and most famous *Tyrannosaurus rex* skeleton."

The museum's gift shops were treasures in themselves, and we gave them equal time, just browsing.

Tam was determined to cram as much life into each day as she possibly could. She didn't want to miss seeing and tasting and experiencing everything this place had to offer. She didn't want to waste even one second. It didn't matter that she was exhausted most of the time; she could give in and rest when we returned home.

Between our treks to see area attractions, Tam was still trying to work for Proteome, reviewing new medical research papers and entering pertinent information on their database via the Internet. My friend Eloisa Brown had loaned Tammy her laptop computer to use on the trip. And I was working on a business article for the *Albuquerque Journal*. Tammy sat at the computer at the little counter in the kitchenette, and I sat in a chair, writing my story out in longhand. Once I had it finished, I tried to type it out on the laptop so I could send it in by e-mail. But I worked on an iMac at home; I had no idea how to use the word-processing program on the laptop. I just assumed that if you could use one program, you could probably use any of them. Not so! I couldn't, anyway. So Tammy gave me a crash course in the fine points of using Microsoft Word on the laptop computer. Eventually I got the hang of it and sent the story on its way.

With that marvelous little laptop and the wonders of e-mail, we kept up with the news from home and we let people there know what was going on with us. The first thing in the morning, even before breakfast, Tam checked her e-mail. As soon as we returned from our forays, she checked e-mail. She checked it the last thing at night before we went to bed. She loved all the news and words of encouragement. Especially those from Richard.

Besides his chatty notes with news and gossip, Richard wrote poetry for her. The funny ones she read to me. Others she read, then grinned and blushed but didn't share them with me. I so very much wanted to peek at those missives from Richard, but I could never get to the computer without Tammy around to catch me.

From our third-floor window, we watched the snow fall. We could see the fat flakes swirl and dance in the light cast by the streetlight below. Almost as soon as the first flakes hit the ground, dump trucks loaded with salt and sand and equipped with snow blades on front began scurrying up and down the road, clearing away the snow accumulation while scattering salt on the roadways. A pickup truck with a snow blade on it zipped around the parking lot of the hotel, clearing the snow away as it fell. From our vantage point, they looked like a bunch of agitated ants. At home in New Mexico, a couple of inches of snow have a major impact—schools are closed and traffic comes to a standstill. But here traffic zoomed on the roads and highways as usual; a little thing like snow didn't get in the way of the daily business of life.

Day by day, Tammy seemed to get stronger, and the gray, sick look gradually faded. The pain went away, and she just looked healthier. Even her hair started to grow back. She didn't have to draw her eyebrows on with an eyebrow pencil anymore. They came back in dark brown, but the hair on her head was like transparent peach fuzz. It was hard to tell if it was going to be dark again or salt-and-pepper or even white. Whatever its eventual color, she was just glad to have it back, I think. But she began to feel very tired as the anticipated side effects of the radiation set in.

From Tammy's journal:

January 25, 2002

I've been here almost three weeks, and I'm a little over halfway with the radiation. It's much easier than the chemo was. I get a little nauseous but not too bad. This week the doc says I may get diarrhea, which will be a drag if it happens, but it will be temporary.

My hair is starting to come back! Being bald is very chilly, so the hair will come in handy. It's been warmer than usual this winter in Illinois, but it's still plenty cool for me.

I borrowed a laptop from my mom's friend so I can e-mail my buddies and do some database work. I can get my e-mail at my regular address, but I forgot to bring a list of addresses. No problem, though, my friends are sending me e-mails anyway.

I'll be happy to get back to Albuquerque and real life. But this trip has been like a vacation. Mom and I have just had the best time eating out and poking around all the museums in downtown Chicago.

Diarrhea was expected; nausea wasn't. She didn't have problems with diarrhea until much later, but nausea was a disagreeable side effect she coped with for the remainder of our stay.

Homesickness began to nibble at Tam's euphoria. She was very glad we came, but the crushing fatigue was defeating her willpower. She was too tired for much sightseeing, and she missed seeing the people she loved at home.

Her energy gave out at a handy time; it was cheaper to stay in the hotel than to take in the sights. Our funds were running out. I didn't want Tam to go home feeling that we had missed the opportunity to really see and enjoy the Chicago area. But I didn't want to spend all our resources and get into real financial trouble either. The gas and the admission fees and the cost of eating at restaurants were adding up much faster than I anticipated. I didn't tell Tam about my concerns; she had enough to worry about.

We began to explore the towns nearby so we could still see the area without spending anything except the gas to get there, and if Tam was really tired, we just drove—we didn't even get out of the car.

Less than a mile from our hotel, we found a great place to pause and eat. It was a combined bakery and sandwich shop that served, among other things, hot homemade soup in a hollowed-out, personal-sized, crusty loaf of French bread. When we were tired or homesick or simply in the mood for it, we sat in a booth beside the large window and watched the snow fall as we each savored hot clam chowder or other fresh soup in its own bread bowl. It was the greatest comfort food ever.

Sometimes we went to the movies in the afternoon; we saw the first *Harry Potter* movie there and loved it. Or we simply walked around the pond on the hotel grounds and watched the snow geese. One weekend, our big adventure was a trek to the Morton Arboretum to see an ice sculpture show. It was a display of fantastic crystal-clear creations fashioned with chainsaws from large blocks of ice. Some of the ice sculptures were in the process of being carved as we watched. Amazing!

One night, we took in a poetry slam at the Ramsey Auditorium in Wilson Hall on the Fermi grounds. Typical of the paradoxical nature of the place, Ramsey Auditorium was an elegant theater with plush seats and red carpet located on the lower level of the building. To get there, we walked down a red carpeted aisle with heavy machinery clanking on either side.

The poetry slam was not at all what I expected. I probably wouldn't have gone, but as with many things these days, Tammy was curious. She wanted to see just what it was all about. Comparing this to what I expected would have been like comparing Louie Armstrong to Beethoven. These people didn't just read their poetry; they performed it. People in the audience didn't just watch; they were enthralled. During one segment of the program, members of the audience were invited to perform their own poetry. We were surprised at just how many people had brought their own poetry, prepared to participate.

Tam and I went from being eager tourists to being weary travelers. We wanted to go home. Chicago was exciting and Fermi was still the fount of hope, but we were ready to go home and get back to our real lives—to familiar surroundings and homemade meals and friends dropping by.

-8-

On Tammy's good days, we began browsing through the shops in the nearby towns—Aurora, Naperville, St. Charles, Geneva, Batavia—looking for gifts for friends and family back home.

Each town had a strip of shops along its main street—gift shops, bead shops, T-shirt shops, all sorts of places to buy goodies to take back home with us. We were looking for really neat things, unique things that didn't cost much.

"Classy junk, not cheap junk," Tammy said.

In the process, we found a delightful little bookstore in St. Charles. An historic old house had been converted into the Town House Books and Cafe. The wooden floors creaked, dark wood paneling cloaked the walls, and a fire crackled in a potbellied stove. It smelled of woodsmoke and books. Shelves lined with books filled every room. Even the large porch across the front of the house had been glassed in to provide space for yet more books.

We found familiar books, new books, old books, fascinating books, fun books. It became an almost-regular haunt after Tammy's nuke sessions at Fermilab. After browsing and sometimes buying, we ambled into the café room for a cup of tea and sometimes a pastry before heading back to our hotel room.

By the time we were ready to start making serious plans to go back home, we had collected a nice little stash of booty to take back with us—T-shirts and baseball caps and puzzles from the Fermilab gift shop; small dragonfly ornaments and snail fossil magnets from the Morton Arboretum gift shop; elaborate, exotic beads and knickknacks from other gift shops; and of course, books. We kept in mind the logistics of getting things home as we collected each item, selecting things that were relatively small and packable. But when they were all piled together on the bed, it was obvious we had gone a bit overboard.

No problem.

We packed it all into a couple of cartons and mailed them home. Now all we had to do was get through the time left before we could go home.

Most of the other patients at Fermi were on a schedule similar to Tammy's. Of course, everybody went on the same days of the week because the beam was only available three days a week; beam time was scheduled to synchronize with Fermi research projects. Most patients had begun their series of treatments about the same time as Tam and expected to finish at about the same time. Consequently, we developed almost a sense of family with the patients and the people who accompanied them, as well as the staff working there, in a fairly short time. As Tammy noted, everybody there had a story. By the time they got there, they were all rejects from the usual treatment protocols. And apparently the technicians and nurses and doctors there didn't go along with the "don't get emotionally involved" rule.

There was the man who came with an advanced case of prostate cancer, frightened and withdrawn when we first saw him; he became much more relaxed and outgoing as his symptoms receded, and hope returned. By the time he went home, all traces of his cancer were gone, at least for the time being, and he was almost giddy.

And there was the middle-aged woman whose daughter and husband brought her in a wheelchair laden with oxygen tanks and panic. Her breast cancer had metastasized and had wrapped itself around her esophagus and invaded her chest cavity, collapsing a lung in the process.

Her oncologist had given her no more than three or four days before the cancer would take her life. Her daughter had found Fermi on the Internet, so she called them on the phone, and the next day, the woman, her husband, and her daughter drove from their home in Minnesota to Fermi. After three treatments, her tumors had become small enough that her lung reinflated, buying her at least a little more time.

Then there was Missy, a young woman perhaps a little older than Tammy who was there because her ovarian cancer had metastasized to her spine. She had steel-gray hair, dark eyebrows, and a wicked sense of humor. She could still walk, but her gait was stiff and cautious, very much like Tammy's.

Her husband had stayed behind with their thirteen-year-old daughter. She seemed to worry about them and their well-being in her absence much more than she did about her own circumstances. She too had been given only a short time to live. She fully expected to lose her fight with cancer, and she was making long-term plans to make life easier for her daughter and her husband after her death. But maybe, just maybe, Fermi could buy her some time. And maybe, just maybe, there was a tiny chance that she might survive. She too had learned about Fermi and their neutron therapy on the Internet. She had taken the initiative to gather all the necessary referrals and make all the arrangements and get herself there on her own, without help from anybody else. After just a few treatments, her skin color improved, the pain relaxed its grip on her spine, and her face let go of its constant grimace.

Another miracle. They all were, one way or another. For some of them, cancer was permanently eradicated; for the rest, neutrons extended their lives a bit longer.

Missy was from out of state, but she stayed with friends in West Chicago while undergoing treatment at Fermi. One weekend, Missy and her friend Joan invited Tammy and me to Joan's house for Sunday dinner.

It seemed like an eternity since we had been inside a real home. At the dinner table with Missy, Joan, and her husband, Lee, we all talked as if we had known each other for years. We laughed and ate roast beef and salad and talked some more. I hadn't realized how much I missed ordinary dinner-table conversation with an ordinary family in an ordinary house.

Our lives had come to revolve around Fermi and Tammy's treatments there. Tammy and I had thoroughly enjoyed our adventures as tourists in Chicago between her treatments—the museums and the restaurants and the wonderful places to see—but now we were ready to go home.

On Tam's January 29 session, one of her last before we headed back home, Dr. Shafer had a medical student with him.

"Angiosarcoma is relatively rare," he told the student. "The average oncologist sees only one or two in his career. We see lots more because we treat sarcomas. They look benign, but they don't act benign. Tammy's problem with getting a diagnosis is typical.

"Tammy had aggressive chemo that was effective in shutting her tumors down for now, but they often come back chemo resistant. So we're radiating them all. We're treating all known tumors, hoping that the neutrons will take care of all tumor activity and that any cells that got loose were taken care of with chemo."

Good! That's what we were hoping too.

After examining Tammy and asking her a series of questions about how she was faring with the radiation, he determined that her bowels were fine, her urine was fine, her appetite was declining, her nausea was getting a little better, her pain level was about the same, and there was no weakness in her leg.

"You're doing very well," he told her. "Your treatment is aggressive, but not super aggressive. We don't want to jeopardize your quality of life. With the bowel involved, we don't want excessive scarring, especially since you've had radiation before."

We went to our favorite lunchtime haunt for soup-in-a-bread-bowl and watched snowflakes pile up on the windowsill outside. Tammy talked about what she wanted to do when we got back home, mostly small, ordinary things—have her car washed and waxed or take Cindy and Terri out for lunch and a movie. She also wanted to write an article for a scientific journal about Fermilab and their use of neutron radiation to treat cancer. It was the first time in a very long time that she had talked about future plans at all. Perhaps she was beginning to think that she might actually have a future.

Her next trek to Fermi was routine, but a little problem surfaced after her blood test at the following one.

"Your white counts are way down," the nurse on duty said. "You've got to rest, no goofing around till they come back up. We'll send you to St. Joe's for Neupogen—that should speed things up."

Tammy saw Dr. Shafer a few minutes later. "You'll get Neupogen today, maybe you can get another dose tomorrow. Your white counts are 1.7. That's really strange. The chemo probably knocked it down, and the marrow is not responsive.

We're (neutron radiation) the straw that broke the camel's back. We'll get you Neupogen—we don't want you to get into trouble."

Then he questioned her closely. Was she having pain? It was much better. Did she still need pain meds? No. Excellent! Nausea? Manageable, so long as she kept food in her stomach. Urination? Okay. Bowel? Loose. Use Imodium.

"We're belt-and-suspenders people," he said. "We tend to go overboard, but we have to. We're treating shallow, it shouldn't affect the marrow. But lots of blood vessels pass through that area, so the blood is getting radiated and it isn't getting replenished from the marrow. The marrow is probably still suppressed from the chemo."

Okay, a small setback. Nothing we couldn't cope with. Tammy's spirits and mine were undaunted.

The Neupogen finally kicked in, and Tammy's white counts came up—not as much as Shafer would have liked, but they came up.

We arranged an interview with Dr. Arlene Lennox, the director of the Neutron Therapy Facility at Fermi, so Tammy could gather the information to write an article for a scientific journal and I could gather information for a potential article for a magazine.

Dr. Lennox (Arlene to us, as well as to the other patients and their families) was a no-nonsense but friendly woman in her late forties or early fifties. She wore not suits or fancy clothes but slacks, nice tops, and comfortable shoes—clothes she could move and work in. She looked like someone whose job was to get her hands dirty if necessary to keep things running smoothly—not what I expected of an executive. And though she always seemed to be on her way to an urgent task somewhere, she took time to stop and chat with each patient. Her words weren't generic—no "How are you?" without staying long enough for an answer, no "Nice day, isn't it?" as she walked away. She knew each patient by name, and she knew their medical history, so her comments were specific. She wasn't just "making nice"; she really cared.

She gave us more than an hour of her time and answered all our questions without hesitation. She is a physicist, not a medical doctor, but her position at the Neutron Therapy Facility wasn't just a job—it was her passion.

ABOUT THE NEUTRON THERAPY FACILITY AT FERMILAB

"When we started research in 1976, nobody knew if this therapy was going to work or not," Lennox said, "so those first patients were pretty much all terminal. All those patients who came in those first ten years were essentially people who had no other options, and the very early ones we did were people that we considered to be terminal."

Even so, their overall success rate with the three thousand one hundred or so patients they had treated so far was something like 58 percent, she said.

She told us about a patient who was treated there in 1976 for a salivary gland tumor. In September 2001, he came back to help celebrate at the facility's twenty-fifth anniversary party.

Despite their success, funding is a continuing problem. For the first ten years, they were funded by the National Cancer Institute to carry out research to see if neutron therapy truly is a viable option for treating difficult cancers. After the ten-year research period was over, the National Cancer Institute expected the Neutron Therapy Facility to shut down since Fermilab was a physics lab, not a medical facility. They expected hospitals that were also doing research with neutrons to pick up the treatment.

"We had better results than most of these hospitals," Lennox said, "because our physics machine was a higher-energy machine with a better dose rate and better penetration than the things they had in their hospitals. So our doctors wanted to continue.

"I think one of the reasons that our treatments here did better than the other hospitals in the '70s and '80s was that, being a physics lab, we had sophisticated computer programs that the hospitals didn't have. We had access to accelerator experts who made this accelerator run routinely. I've been here seventeen years now, and there's only been maybe three days that we had to cancel treatment because something was really broken and we needed to get it fixed."

In 1985, they approached Medicare to establish billing codes and to get them to pay for treatment. Medicare finally agreed. But insurance companies were reluctant to follow suit. They assumed that since the treatment was being done at Fermilab, the government was paying for it. It wasn't. So the NTF had to cut staff, and the two physicians who had been the principal investigators in the research worked on for free.

More insurance companies recognize the validity of the treatment now, and NTF has partnered with other medical facilities, first with St. Joseph's Hospital (Provena) and then with the University of Illinois Medical School. Many, if not most, of NTF's patients learn about the facility's existence from their website.

"These days, patients have to be their own advocates if they want decent medical care," Lennox said.

Still, even though neutrons have proven their merit in treating intractable cancers, the Neutron Therapy Facility continues to struggle for adequate funding. Arlene Lennox has, of necessity, come to spend much of her time writing grants and scrounging for money, in addition to her chores as director and physicist. She refuses to let NTF die for lack of funding.

Tammy had her three radiation sessions the next week—the last one on Friday, as usual. The next day, February 9, we went home. Two days later, I came down with the flu, but thank heavens Tammy didn't get it.

-9-

$\mathcal{F}$ebruary 2002 was a grand month! It was so good to be home. The very air sparked with relief and joy and hope. It had been such a close call for Tam, but now she just might survive after all.

She was glad to be back in her own apartment and to be able to drive her own car by herself, wherever and whenever she wanted. And she was glad to see Richard again. He had gotten her a warm ski jacket to wear in Chicago. Then, worrying that it might not be warm enough, at the last minute, he had loaned her his own full-length down coat. It was never cold enough while we were there for her to wear the coat, but she lugged it around with her everywhere we went just the same, almost as if it were a security blanket. Richard came to see her almost as soon as she first walked in the door of her apartment after we got home. She reluctantly gave him back his down coat, unworn but much traveled.

Richard, as well as the rest of Tammy's friends, wanted to know all about her adventures in Chicago, and she delighted in telling them. She made the scary times, the times when we got lost or overwhelmed by the big, unfamiliar city, sound funny and exciting. The whole thing, as she recounted it, was a wildly successful pleasure trip, with her treatment at Fermi at the heart of it.

Dave Bice, who had been her mentor when she worked as a postdoctoral fellow at the Lovelace Respiratory Research Institute in Albuquerque, owned a small airplane.

One Sunday morning, he took her up on a flight over the Sandia and Manzano Mountains and along the Rio Grande river basin.

She was delighted! She couldn't stop talking about the views from the air and the exhilaration she felt riding so high above the ground in the tiny plane.

On February 18, after months of having it in place, the catheter in her chest was removed. No more chemo now. She wasn't allowed to swim while the catheter was in place because the risk of infection was too great, but she wasted no time getting back into the swimming pool again once it was out. It had been entirely too long since she had been in the water.

She was due to have a series of follow-up scans in May, after her bones had a chance to heal from the radiation. But by late March, she started having pain in her back again. Dr. Tarnower said it could be caused by the bones shifting as the tumors in her spine shrunk, but she wanted Tam to have her scans early, just to be sure. The scan's results weren't good.

Like an old B movie, voices tumbled around in my head, voices once heard and now recalled. "This is not good." "We can give you hope." "People with more disease activity than yours have beaten this thing." "I finally feel like I have a future to plan for." "Don't worry, we'll get the money. Whatever it takes, we'll do it." "You're not a dead cat . . . you're not a dead cat . . . you're not a dead cat."

Tammy kept saying she was so sorry as though it was her fault that this thing was back again. I tried to reassure her, but it didn't help. She said she remembered the cat that a friend gave her. The cat got sick, and Tam said she spent a small fortune in veterinary bills for the poor thing, but she ended up with a dead cat anyway.

"Well, you're not a dead cat," I said. She laughed.

"Okay, just keep reminding me I'm not a dead cat, not yet anyway."

The phrase became one of those silly things you say to break tension, a secret code that was nonsense to anyone but the two of us.

I knew I'd feel the pain soon, but for the moment, I felt detached. I couldn't allow myself to cry yet. I had to keep it together just a little bit longer. Tammy was trying to be calm and alert, but she was trembling—her shoulders were trembling, her hands were shaking almost uncontrollably, and even her voice was quivering. I had to hold it together for her. I had to keep her upright and alert until we could get out of that place.

The surgeon came in and asked questions and gently prodded and felt and looked at Tam's body, sizing up this new horror. She could find only the one lump, just under the skin a little above the back of Tam's left knee and just under the scar from her first cancer surgery in 1998. It was about the size of an egg or a golf ball, and it was hard and warmer than the surrounding skin. We didn't know that it was another sarcoma, but the circumstantial evidence was overwhelming. Tammy weighed 142 pounds when we got back from Chicago; she weighed 135 now. Her six-foot-tall frame was beginning to look a bit gaunt. Her hemoglobin counts were low when we first got back, but they came up, then began to drop again and drop and drop and drop. And that hot, hard lump looked just like the first one on her left buttock in 1998.

The surgeon wanted to take an incision biopsy before determining a course of action. Tam asked her how many sarcomas she had dealt with, and she said none, not for a very long time.

The thing is, angiosarcomas have some really nasty habits. If they're cut, they bleed. They gush, and it's almost impossible to staunch the flow of blood. And if they're cut but not removed, they get angry and their growth accelerates dramatically. This lump was already growing alarmingly fast—it had grown to golf-ball size in less than a week. Tammy had found it while she was shaving her legs. She was so delighted to have hair on her legs again that she liked to take her time shaving. The last time she had shaved, less than a week before, there was nothing there that she could feel.

Tam was to have an MRI on Thursday, April 11. In the meantime, Tam's doctors in Albuquerque planned to consult with specialists who had experience dealing with sarcomas at comprehensive cancer centers in Tucson, Houston, and Boston.

Fate has a cruel sense of humor. Tam had just gotten the results of her first follow-up bone scan since we left Chicago, and her spine was clear, with no sign of disease activity in her bones.

With the discovery of this new lump, Dr. Tarnower called Fermilab to see if she could go back for more neutron radiation. No, she could not, because this new tumor site was radiated in 1998, and it couldn't be radiated again.

As we waited for her to be taken in for the MRI, a tear slid down Tam's cheek, but her face looked perfectly calm. No sobs, no sniffing. Just a solitary tear sliding down her cheek to her chin, where it dripped away. I said nothing, and she said nothing; we both pretended the tear didn't exist.

Once the MRI was finished, there was nothing to do but wait for the results. Outside in the sunshine once more, I asked her why she was so very sad. What was wrong? Why was she crying?

"Nothing. Everything is just fi—" Then she stopped in midsentence and said, "Richard is thinking of going back to his ex-wife so he can see his kids more."

The MRI found yet another tumor on her leg, more to the front of her thigh and above the one she could feel. Something had to be done soon. Tarnower told her to go home and take it easy. She would do some research to find out what to do next.

Tammy was devastated, then she got angry—again.

She didn't have time to wait for her busy oncologist to do more research. She went home and did it herself. As Dr. Redman (she didn't explain that she was a PhD, not an MD), she didn't have to go through the layers and layers of invisible barriers that keep ordinary people from getting answers. She got right through to the people who could tell her what she wanted to know.

The logistics of traveling to Boston would take too much time. She wanted to go to MD Anderson in Houston, but they told her they couldn't see her until the end of May—nearly two months away—and then just for an evaluation, not for treatment. But her tumor was growing too fast to wait that long. That left the University of Arizona Cancer Center, and all three of the doctors that she had seen there before—Dr. Lobell, Dr. Stea, and Dr. Warneke—shuffled their schedules so they could see her three days later.

They decided against additional chemo unless more tumors popped up. It looked like these tumors were still encapsulated; they had not yet sent tentacles into the surrounding tissue. Tam's team of three heroes agreed that surgery to remove the tumors would be the best course of action. It would require two incisions and the removal of some muscle, but they would do their best to retain the function of her leg.

They also wanted to try a new procedure called brachytherapy. Five or six catheters would be implanted around each incision, and once a day for a week beginning four to five days after the surgery, wires would be inserted into the catheters to deliver high-dose radiation directly to the area around the tumor sites, hopefully without damage to healthy tissue. Tammy's would be the first sarcoma they had treated with brachytherapy.

Of course, there would be a fifty-fifty chance that the incision would dehisce, or split open, as a result of the radiation, Dr. Stea said. No problem. After what Tam had been through, a 50 percent chance sounded pretty good. She would be in the 50 percent to come through the procedure unscathed, we were certain.

Dr. Lobell said that if the cancer came back yet again, there were some really promising new drugs almost ready for clinical trials, and Tammy would be eligible to take part in one. Once again, these people sent us on our way with renewed hope. No guarantees but hope. Tammy might still have a slim chance.

The specter of money problems began to haunt me. Even with the special rates for lodging arranged by the cancer center, the costs added up. The travel and the food and the medical co-pays and incidental living expenses had depleted our money stash. That was irrelevant, really, because our whole family was determined that Tammy would have whatever was necessary for her to survive this thing.

It was perverse good fortune for us that right about that time, credit card companies were doing their utmost to convince people to borrow more and more money. Interest rates were fairly low, and every time we used a credit card, it seemed, the company raised our spending limit to entice us to spend even more. Great! That's how we would pay for Tam's care for as long as we could get away with it. I knew full well that we were being seduced into insurmountable debt.

Fine, I thought. *We'll let them pay for as many expenses as we need and let them worry about getting their money back from us after this is over. We cannot afford this—they know we cannot afford this—and still they urge us to charge. We'll deal with the consequences when Tam's fight is over, and if they get shafted, so be it.*

In addition to having three credit cards with ever-expanding spending limits, one credit card company offered us a conventional loan of $15,000 to be paid back at 6 percent interest over six years. We could cope with that with a clear conscience, so we applied for and obtained the loan. Now we could make plans for Tam's next surgery and treatment and not worry about how we were going to pay for them.

Soon after our return to Albuquerque and before we went back to Tucson for this next surgery, Tammy got a call from TVI, the community college where she had taught biology labs one summer. They wanted her to come back and teach in the fall. She told them what was going on with her cancer, but they asked her to come in and fill out the paperwork anyway. They said she could always back out if her medical problems were still an issue.

She was elated! Not only did she have a tiny chance at survival still, she also had a job to plan for—and a future.

It was a warm spring, and Tammy really wanted to plant a garden, but since she lived in an apartment, she had nowhere to put it. Cindy, however, had a large backyard that was mostly wild. She offered to share some of her backyard with Tammy for a garden, and Tammy joyfully took her up on the offer. Cindy hauled in bales of straw and put them in a row around the perimeter of the future garden to delineate it from the rest of the yard and to protect the new seedlings somewhat from the relentless New Mexico spring winds until they could grow strong enough to cope with them on their own.

Cindy did the digging and the heavy work while Tammy planned where to place the seeds and baby plants and helped with the planting. They didn't plant things in rows but in the familiar double-helix patterns. Tomatoes and basils twined around marigolds and cosmos. Eggplants, cantaloupes, watermelons, and peppers framed the helix. As the seeds came up and the tiny plants started to grow, there were way too many plants for the space, but they couldn't bear to pull a single one. But it all seemed to work out somehow. Rabbits got some of the plants, but the neighborhood cats chased most of the rabbits away. Bugs got after some of them, but birds got after the bugs. And so it went, with their topsy-turvy garden thriving. It produced several gallons of tomatoes a day. The tomatoes were passed on to friends and family, with the extras made into soup to freeze for winter.

Sometimes on warm summer evenings, they put bath towels on top of the straw bales and stretched out on them, enjoying the smells and the warm moist air from the garden and looking for falling stars.

Tam and I returned to Tucson on Monday, May 6, for her preop exam. Wayne stayed home to keep things in order there. Again she saw all three doctors—Dr. Lobell, Dr. Warneke, and Dr. Stea. They treated her like a colleague almost—someone that they truly cared about.

On Tuesday, May 7, her surgery was preceded by a CT scan at 10:00 a.m. to locate the exact position of the second tumor and to insert a small hooked wire to mark it for the surgeon.

The surgery got underway at 1:30 p.m. It was expected to take a couple of hours since there would be two large incisions, and they wanted to biopsy the second tumor to confirm that it was malignant (it was) before closing the incision.

I made my way to the waiting room after they wheeled Tammy to the operating room. Wayne's sister, Evie, got there about the same time I did. She had made the two-hour drive from her home in Gilbert to keep me company while I waited.

We sat and talked and waited. We talked about ordinary, everyday things, and time passed. Finally, just before five o'clock, Dr. Warneke came out to tell us about Tam's surgery. I think Evie was glad to be there to hear the report firsthand, and I was very glad to have her there.

Both tumors were indeed fairly well encapsulated, not yet extended into the surrounding tissue. (Good news!) They removed some of the muscle around the little one and some muscle and quite a bit of skin with the larger one.

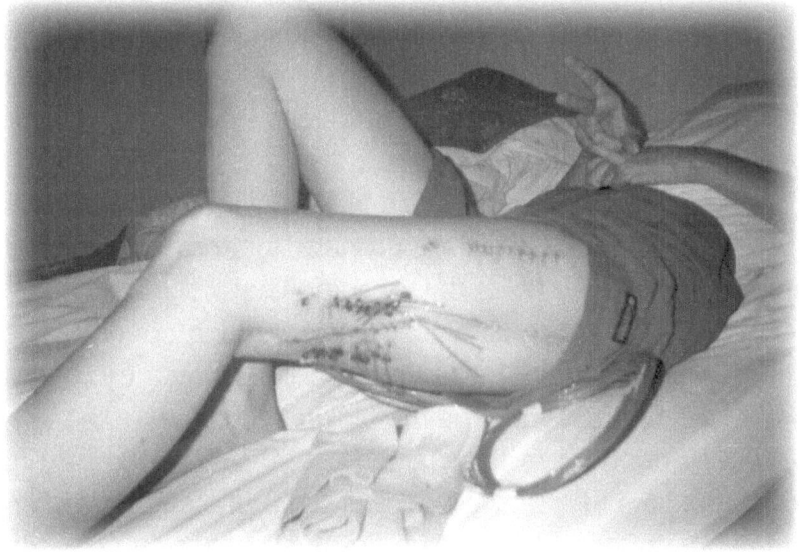

Tam's incisions with the catheters implanted for brachytherapy.

Warneke said that even with the hooked-wire marker, he had a hard time finding the smaller tumor. He was fairly sure he got clean margins with no cancer cells left behind, but the pathology people would have to examine it to be sure. Nine catheters were implanted in the larger incision. None were implanted in the incision for the smaller tumor because they didn't think it was necessary. Besides, that area had already been irradiated; more radiation would do more harm than good.

When Warneke was finished talking to us, Evie headed home and I waited for Tam to come out of the recovery room. She was taken up to her room at about 7:00 p.m., very groggy but lucid and cheerful.

The next day, Tam was discharged from the hospital, still in pain and unable to walk, but she felt better back at our apartment. She could drink all the water she wanted whenever she wanted, and finally she could eat. First, just the broth from chicken ramen, then macaroni and cheese and applesauce—not terribly nutritious, but that was her comfort food of choice.

Tam had an appointment at 11:00 a.m. at the University of Arizona Cancer Center to prepare for the radiation, but communications were derailed somewhere along the line, and nobody in Dr. Stea's office knew anything about it. They asked us to stay until 1:00 p.m., and they would try to work Tam in. We sat and watched the clown fish cavort in the large saltwater aquarium in the waiting room. We leafed through old magazines. I drank cup after cup of coffee from the communal coffee pot, and Tam drank cup after cup of water. Finally, at 1:30 p.m., they called her name and wheeled her into an examination room via wheelchair with crutches as a backup. She didn't want to be stranded in a wheelchair; she wanted to be able to go where she wanted. Whether a wheelchair would fit or not, she could use the crutches if she had to.

Evie and her daughter, Gail (who was more like a sister than a cousin to Tam and Terri), were planning to be at our apartment by 2:30 p.m., but it was after 3:30 p.m. before we left the exam room. All the preliminary work had been done to get the radiation treatments underway beginning the next Wednesday, May 15. Tammy would have two radiation sessions a day, one at 9:00 a.m. and one at 3:00 p.m., for three consecutive days. They had changed the timing, I think, because they had waited a few days longer than originally planned to let her leg heal before starting the radiation, but they didn't want to make us have to stay away from home any longer than absolutely necessary.

When we returned to our apartment, Evie and Gail were waiting for us. They had brought Tammy a bouquet of flowers. We all went inside, and Tam noodled her way to the couch on the crutches, stretched out, and held court for the next hour or so as Evie and Gail updated us on what was happening in the outside world. Lots of laughter, a few tears, and a whole lot of love.

Terri, Cindy, and Wayne called several times a day (thank goodness for cell phones!) to keep up with what was going on with us. Tam and I called them frequently too. When we weren't doing medical things at the cancer center, we were exploring the Tucson area. Most of the places Tammy wanted to see involved walking long distances, but fortunately for her, most of them had wheelchairs available to borrow. Thus we were able to traverse the endless paths at the Arizona-Sonora Desert Museum and the Biosphere 2 Center with no problems. We haunted their gift shops for goodies to give to the people at home. We had developed the knack in Chicago, we were certain, of discerning good junk from, well, tacky junk, so the things we chose would be something the folks at home would treasure, even though we couldn't spend a lot of money on it. Those bright-blue eighteen-inch-long pencils from the Biosphere would be perfect, and they only cost a buck apiece.

On the days when Tam was really tired, we went to the movies where she could rest while she watched the movie. She didn't want to waste the time staying in our room when there was so much to see and to do in Tucson. She was the one who was sick, but I was the one struggling to keep up.

Her shoulder began to ache a day or so after the surgery. When the ache persisted, she asked her doctors about it. They thought it had probably been caused by her being placed in an awkward position or by someone tugging on her arm a bit too hard as they repositioned her during the surgery. No problem. It should go away before long.

When her radiation treatments were all finished, they took the catheters out and we headed home. The doctors told her the incisions would probably take longer to heal than usual because of the radiation.

Wayne and I expected her to stay with us for a week or so, but she stayed only the first night, then she went back to her own apartment. We had our doubts about her negotiating those two flights of stairs to her apartment, but she did it just fine. It took her a while, but she did it.

-10-

$\mathcal{A}$t about nine o'clock in the morning, on June 5, Tammy called and said that when she bent over to tie her shoe, the incision on the back of her leg split open. Could I please come?

When I got there, I could see an opening about two-and-a-half inches long and half-an-inch-or-so deep in the incision. I drove her to the oncologist's office, but nobody there knew what to do about it. Finally, a physician's assistant named Mary Antle put several Steri-Strips on it to hold it closed, then bandaged it. Thank goodness we were scheduled to go back to Tucson for her postsurgery checkup the next week.

Dave Bice flew Tammy and me back to Tucson in his small airplane on Monday, June 10. It was a Piper Comanche four-seater.

I really don't like high places. I don't even climb above the third rung of a ladder—that is as high off the ground as I'll go. I was on the edge of raw, naked panic at the prospect of flying in that tiny plane, while Tammy was giddy with joy. But the ride wasn't nearly as terrifying as I expected, I suppose because the cockpit felt more secure than I thought it would. Dave pointed out landmarks as we flew over. Though we had seen many of them from the car before, they looked very different from above.

When we arrived at the Tucson airport, we were treated like visiting royalty. We climbed out of the plane and walked to an executive lounge to make arrangements to park the plane, stepped over to the next counter and rented a car, walked back outside, climbed into the car, and were on our way. No walking miles and miles across the terminal, no being jostled by huge crowds, no waiting in lines. This was truly the way to fly!

When Dr. Warneke looked at the dehisced (reopened) wound, I saw a brief look of despair cross his face, then he was all business. He said that once the incision had dehisced, it wouldn't grow back together; it would have to heal from the bottom up. They knew, and we knew, from the outset that there was a 50 percent chance of this happening, but both Tam and I had chosen to believe that she would be in the lucky 50 percent that healed. We were wrong.

Dr. Stea and Dr. Lobell came in to look at it. Their eyes filled with sorrow; their voices said this was only a small setback. They showed us how to care for it, then we met Dave Bice and flew back home in his tiny plane. We landed at the Double Eagle Airport, west of Albuquerque, at sunset and were back home by dark.

That dehisced incision became almost like another family member—it was always at the forefront of our attention. Since it was on the back of her thigh, Tammy couldn't reach it to care for it, and that annoyed her no end. Tending it was a major production. I promptly forgot all the instructions they had given us in Tucson, but Terri's training in wound care was a godsend. She carefully wrote out instructions so that I could take care of the incision when she could not. Between us, we made sure it got cleaned and bandaged daily.

First, and often, I washed my hands. If I forgot, Tam reminded me. Then I donned laetrile gloves (I had developed an allergy to latex gloves, as had Terri), unwrapped Tam's leg, and checked the wound to see if it was smelly or hot.

(That would have meant infection had set in, with a whole new set of problems.) I cleaned the wound off gently with a Q-tip, washed it with hydrogen peroxide, and dried it with sterile four-by-four gauze pads. I wiped the edges of the wound with something called Bard to keep them dry, then applied antibiotic ointment to the wound with a clean Q-tip. Next, I wiped the scissor blades with an alcohol wipe, cut a strip of Sorbsan, one inch long, and very carefully packed it into the wound to absorb any discharge. I covered it with Adaptic, then a four-by-four gauze pad, and wrapped the whole thing with Kling bandage and finished off with an elasticized compression bandage. All used bandages and supplies were bagged and disposed promptly.

This had to be done every single day, and before long, I actually got the routine down pat.

Tammy's shoulder continued to hurt, so at her request, Dr. Tarnower ordered an MRI to see what was causing the pain. It showed a sizeable mass under her pectoral muscles, on top of her shoulder bone. Tammy's body just insisted on growing those damned tumors.

We went back to Tucson on Wednesday, June 19. Thursday we went to the University of Arizona Cancer Center. Dr. Lobell was already double-booked, but he said he would work Tam in anyway.

After examining her and looking at the MRI films, he ordered a full-body PET scan to see just what was going on.

"I think we should shrink the tumor before surgery," Dr. Lobell said. "The smaller they are, the better our chances of success. This one is fairly large. Ifosfamide has worked well for us. Angiosarcomas tend to be very responsive. It will depend upon what this thing looks like on a PET scan and on what else is around."

She had the PET scan on Friday afternoon. She wasn't to eat anything beforehand, then just before the scan, she drank a radioactive juice. Since cancer cells take up carbohydrates faster than healthy cells, the cancer cells show up as white areas on the scan.

She finished the scan at 4:00 p.m., and the radiologist said it would take him an hour or so to go over the hundreds of pictures produced by the scan and make his preliminary report. Both Dr. Lobell and Dr. Warneke waited with Tam and me for the results.

The scan showed the mass in her shoulder to be the only real tumor, but there were a couple of other hot spots, one in her spine and one at the incision site on the back of her leg. The doctors said it was possible that they were caused by inflammation, a part of the healing process.

Dr. Lobell wanted Tam to start ultra-high-dose ifosfamide, a treatment that was under study at the cancer center, to shrink this new tumor before having surgery to remove it. Then she would have more radiation. She would have to be hospitalized at the cancer center in Tucson for the chemo.

Since Tam's and Terri's thirty-eighth birthday was Sunday, June 23, she wanted to go home to celebrate it with Terri before starting the new treatment. We were scheduled to return to Tucson so she could begin the chemo on Wednesday, June 26.

On the morning of her birthday, Tam woke up in a really bad mood.

She wanted to go to the High Finance Restaurant at the top of the tram on Sandia Mountain for dinner to celebrate Terri's and her birthday. So that's what we did. But the closer it came to time to go, the grumpier she got. She couldn't decide what to wear. I drove too fast. Wayne was too slow. Nothing was quite right.

We met Cindy and her two girls, Terri and Mark, and Mark's two sisters and his nephew at the base of the tram, then we all boarded and started the fifteen-minute, 2.7-mile ascent up the side of the mountain. There were eleven of us altogether.

The view from the tram as it makes its way up the mountain is usually spectacular, but that day, smoke from forest fires that burned around New Mexico as well as in Arizona and Colorado filled the air; everything was obliterated in a mass of haze.

The haze didn't seem to dampen the spirits of the thirty or so people riding the tram with us, however. They joked and laughed all around us, and their mood was contagious. Soon our group was partaking in the merriment too.

When we got to the restaurant, we had to wait while the staff put three tables together to accommodate our group.

When we were finally seated, Mark's sisters gave Tam and Terri each a huge gift bag filled with dozens of gifts, all with a Scooby Doo (the cartoon dog character) motif on them. There was everything from a video and a CD to caps and coloring books and crayons. In the midst of the chaos of opening the gifts, the waitress took our orders, then Terri and Tammy continued opening their goodies. Tammy's gloom had turned to glee, and she and Terri gaily assumed their roles as co-queens of the day. They wore their Scooby Doo garb, and we all oohed and aahed over their loot.

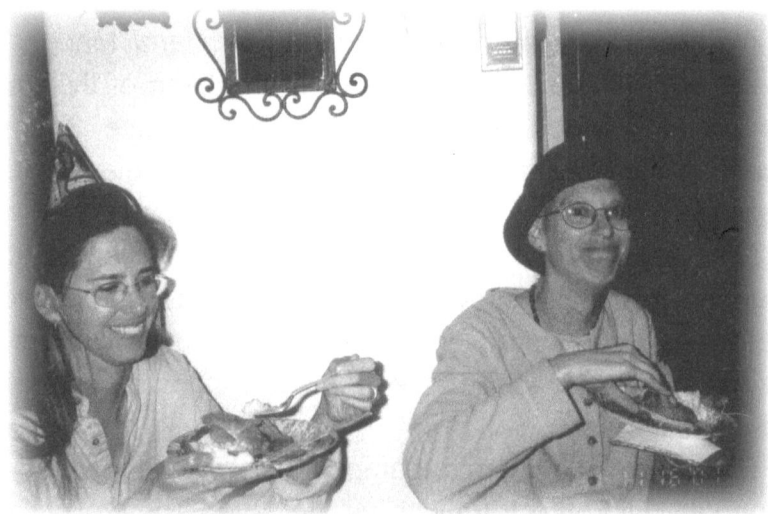

Terri, left and Tammy eating their birthday cake.

While some restaurants use dim lighting or eclectic decor to create ambience, this one had huge windows all around to take full advantage of the views. As the sun went down, the smoky haze turned a bright, glowing orange, swirling around the nearby trees and cliffs while obliterating the view of Albuquerque and the west mesa beyond. It lent a beautiful, soft, ethereal aura to the evening.

We were beginning to get a bit worried before our food was finally served—it had been an hour since the waitress took our orders. The food was great, the service was lousy, and the prices were enough to take my breath away, but we had a grand time. When it was time to go, I started packing the mountains of wrapping paper into bags to take with us. Terri and Tammy both strenuously objected. Instead, with eager assistance from Heather and Chelsea (Cindy's girls) and Ian (Mark's nephew), they stuffed it all under the tables as revenge for being ignored by the waitress. It was the Ts' birthday, after all, so we let them have their way.

On Tuesday, June 25, Tam and I were packed and ready to leave for Tucson when she got a call from Dr. Lobell. Since Tammy had had ifosfamide before, she couldn't have it in the high dosage that he had planned. Surgery and radiation were out because they would do more harm than good. She could get the lower dose of ifosfamide in Albuquerque, so there was no need to go back to Tucson.

Well, we tried. The medical facility in Albuquerque couldn't start the chemo until the following Monday, almost a week later. It was so frustrating! In Albuquerque she was "just one of the masses," as she put it, while in Tucson she was a patient with critical needs and they did their best to take care of her as soon as possible. The difference was probably due to the shortage of doctors in Albuquerque, but meanwhile, her tumor was growing full tilt.

Tam refused to let the situation get her down—or maybe she refused to accept its portent.

"Okay, then, let's get psyched for another battle," she said. "We can't stop the waves, but we can learn to surf."

She planned to have the full chemo regimen—four sessions—and then push to get a referral back to Fermilab in Chicago. Neutron radiation kills angiosarcoma, which conventional radiation doesn't. If she could just get rid of this latest tumor, there were some clinical trials of some really promising drugs coming up that just might give her a chance to beat this thing. One that sounded particularly promising was of a drug that blocked the uptake of protein in cancer cells with no ill effect on healthy cells, thus killing the cancer cells by starvation.

Wayne and I took a line from an old country Western song recorded by Pam Tillis, something about "Swimmin' in da river of de Nial [Nile]" as our motto. We knew Tam's chances looked grim, and denial was the only way we could cope. And maybe she really would find a cure. We did a lot of swimming in that river.

Tammy had her first round of chemo of this latest session on July 1. Shortly afterward, she began to feel much better and even regained some of the range of motion she had lost in her neck and arm.

Tammy insisted on staying in her own apartment, but she didn't feel up to driving just yet, so I drove her in to have blood tests on Friday, July 12. No wonder she felt tired and listless. Normal white cell counts are between 5 and 10—Tam's were 0.6. They promptly gave her a transfusion of two units of blood. She felt much, much better by the time she finally returned home at 4:00 p.m.

Terri got off work at noon and came to spend a couple of hours chatting with Tammy while she was getting the transfusion. Tammy told Terri and me that she had called Crownpoint, a town on the Navajo Nation in the northwest corner of New Mexico renowned for its handwoven rugs. Gallery owners and collectors came from far and wide to the monthly rug auction there. Tam said the next rug auction was Friday evening, July 14. Terri promptly asked her if she wanted to go. She said, "Yes, but not with you guys. I want to go with Richard, if he wants to go. If he doesn't, you two can come with me."

We were not at all offended; we were delighted with her spunk. And what was this about Richard? We thought he was history. Not so. It seems Richard's reunion with his ex-wife didn't come even close to fruition, and he was back in Tam's life. He did indeed want to go. Later, when I asked how things went at the rug auction, she just said, "Oh, just fine!" with a blush and a wide grin.

Not quite a week later, Tammy developed a fever and chills in the night, and since Terri lived much closer to her than we did, she took Tam to the emergency room. Tam was admitted to the hospital with an infection in the dehisced incision. They administered antibiotics intravenously and released her on July 23 with a prescription for an oral antibiotic. They had taken a culture from the infected skin while she was in the hospital, but the results didn't come back until after she was released. The culprit was *Staphylococcus aureus*, but it was resistant to most of the antibiotics. They took an MRI of her leg. The results came back after she had gone home, showing a pocket of infection under the surface of the skin. She was given a prescription for oral vancomycin, the only truly effective antibiotic for her infection.

Soon after Tam was released from the hospital, she had an MRI of her shoulder to see if the tumor had indeed gotten smaller. The MRI process made the tumor really, really angry. Before the MRI, she had stopped taking pain medications altogether, but afterward, she had trouble finding a combination of medications that would control the pain.

The fever persisted, so on July 25, a home health care nurse came to Tammy's home to hook up an IV drip twice a day to deliver the vancomycin. Soon she taught Tammy how to hook up the IV herself. Since Tam had a catheter implanted in her chest, it was no problem for her to do it.

She couldn't start the next round of chemo until the infection was cleared up, and that was estimated to take from two to four weeks. Meanwhile, her shoulder was becoming more painful by the minute, and the left side of her neck was numb, with pain going down her left arm. Frustrated, I sent a fax to Dr. Shafer at Fermilab, explaining what was going on and asking if it would be possible for her to sandwich in neutron therapy before her next chemo session. He called back and said that if we could get there, they would work her in.

When we finally got the results of the MRI, they showed that the tumor in her shoulder had not gotten smaller—it had grown and spread into the head of the humerus, the bone in her upper arm. It was inoperable; it wasn't in a site accessible to conventional radiation, and the one high dose of ifosfamide did nothing but drop her blood counts into the basement and make her sick. They discontinued it. She lost the use of her left arm.

Once again, we boarded a flight to Chicago.

"Get cancer and see the world" had become Tam's motto. There were a number of organizations that helped arrange low-cost transportation to treatment facilities for people who were gravely ill, but they all took several weeks to get the necessary approvals. We simply didn't have the time. Tam bullied me into trying Priceline.com to find cheap airline tickets. I found some on Delta, and we found a relatively inexpensive room at the Hawthorn Suites in Naperville again because of their arrangement with the Neutron Therapy Facility. But prices were much, much higher in August than they had been in January.

Our first trip to Chicago had been great fun; this one was a tortuous ordeal. Tam was in so much pain that her skin was a pale gray, and there was a permanent blanket of sweat on her upper lip. She clinched her teeth to keep from crying out with the slightest bump or jostle. The people at the airport in Albuquerque could see that she needed help, and a porter got her a wheelchair without even being asked. We brought an ice pack for her shoulder to help deaden the pain, but it didn't help much.

However, the people at the security checkpoints all along our journey were not impressed. At each checkpoint, I was waved through, but Tam aroused intense suspicion. I had to take off her shoes, and she had to stand while someone scanned her with a wand apparatus and closely examined the wheelchair. And each time, tears streamed down her face, and she clinched her teeth even tighter with pain.

Because we were traveling subeconomy class, our seats were cramped for Tam's six-foot frame, and we had several stops. The flight attendants were kind, offering to refill Tam's ice bag or to do anything possible to make her more comfortable. But it was a hard, hard trip.

Tam saw Dr. Shafer the next day, and he ordered an MRI of her whole body to see just what was going on.

I waited in the lounge while Tammy went in for the first neutron radiation treatment. I paced the long, narrow room, looking out the windows and drinking cup after cup of coffee while I waited for her. Finally Dr. Shafer asked me to step in back to look at Tam's latest scans.

He pointed to those ominous white areas not only in her shoulder this time but also up and down her spine, from just above where she had had neutron radiation the last time up to the base of her skull. Unchecked, those tumors were likely to make her a quadriplegic very, very soon.

"This isn't good, it isn't good," he said. Those damned words again, almost word for word what Dr. Tarnower had said nearly a year earlier.

"She's not going to make it," he said. "We have to shift our focus to palliation. That's the best we can do."

Palliation—such an innocuous-sounding word, a polite word that means changing the battle plan from vanquishing the enemy to making the enemy's win as painless as possible. Cancer had won. Now pain was the enemy. *Palliative*—a soft word to relieve the impact of the truth, much better than the word *death*, but an ugly word just the same.

Dr. Shafer invited me to stay in the darkened room while Tammy had her treatment and while he pored over the films from her scans again. It was a most humane offer. I cried silently in the dark, away from curious eyes. He asked if he should tell Tam or if I wanted to tell her. I told him I thought she would want to hear the details from him.

When Tam got back to the waiting room after her treatment, I went out to join her. Dr. Shafer said he'd be out to talk to her in a few minutes. She asked what he had told me. I could think of no way to soften the harsh truth, so I repeated what he had said, that she wasn't going to make it. "You're toast, hon."

Then he came out and gave her the details of the scan results and very gently told her she wasn't going to win this battle. They would nuke all the tumors they could and still leave her with enough healthy bone marrow to produce blood cells. But new tumors would continue to develop.

She seemed to step out of her role as patient and step into her scientist persona, asking him detailed, technical questions about her situation. Her speech did not falter; she did not cry. She just wanted to know the truth, all of it.

"The angiosarcoma cells are elusive and incredibly fast-growing," he said. "It's as if we're trying to trap water in a sieve."

On the way home, we stopped at our favorite eatery, and we each had homemade soup in a hollowed-out bread bowl even though it was a hot August day. Tam was quiet for a long, long time. Finally she said, "I prefer denial. I'm not going to just give up, not without a fight."

I agreed to go along with whatever she wanted to do. Though we both knew better, we went on as though she still had a chance, as though she still had viable options.

The wound, the incision that had split apart, was finally beginning to fill in, ever so slowly. Her hair, which had grown back thick and curly after she lost it with the first chemo regimen, was about an inch long when it abruptly fell out again, roughly three weeks after she started the second series of chemo treatments. She was left with two tufts of hair, one on each side of her forehead, and soft, downy fuzz on the rest of her head. She pulled out her wacky bandannas and hats to wear again.

When we came to Chicago this time, Terri was afraid she would never see Tam alive again. Endless phone calls and e-mails helped, but they weren't the same as seeing for herself just how Tammy was faring.

Somehow Cindy convinced the people at her church to donate enough money to buy a round-trip plane ticket for Terri to fly to Chicago and spend a long weekend with Tam. Terri arrived in Chicago on a Thursday evening. She was anxious to go with Tammy to Fermi for her appointment the next morning. She wanted to see for herself just what they were doing to her twin sister.

The people there were happy to show her once they got over the shock of seeing someone who looked just like Tammy, only with hair. Brian, the technician who administered Tammy's treatment, took the time to give Terri a tour of the treatment facilities. She was even allowed in the treatment room / freight elevator as Brian positioned Tammy for her treatment, then she watched from the control area as the treatment room was lowered into the beam line and Tam's tumors were bombarded with radiation.

Afterward, Tam and I took Terri to our favorite eatery to have clam chowder in a bread bowl. We all needed comfort food.

That afternoon, Tammy developed a high fever. I put in a frantic call to Dr. Shafer, then I dashed to Walgreens to pick up a prescription for antibiotics. Terri sponged her off with a cool washcloth, then sat beside the bed and held her hand. I think Terri was glad to be there to see firsthand what Tammy was going through, and I know Tammy was relieved to have her there.

The next morning, Tam felt weak but better. She and Terri walked around the pond on the hotel grounds and talked. Sometimes they paused to sit on one of the benches beside the path around the pond so Tam could rest a bit before they continued their stroll. Finally they came back to our room and talked for hours while I ran errands, buying groceries and supplies. On Sunday, Terri took the limo back to the airport and flew home to New Mexico, a world away.

This time we didn't drive long distances to take in the sights; it was just too miserable for Tam. She was in so much pain when she first started the neutron radiation treatments that it was difficult for her to tolerate the treatment positions, even with an IV morphine drip. But the pain in her shoulder began to ease up a bit with the neutron radiation, so we explored the grounds at Fermilab. She wanted to see the buffalo herd again, and she wanted to walk in the lush green meadows. They were bright with wildflowers—asters and Queen Anne's lace and goldenrod. She picked a small bouquet of flowers, and when we returned to our room, she carefully placed some of them between layers of paper towels and pressed them between the pages of her journal. They're still there.

Friends and family called often to see how Tam was doing. I had promised Tammy to keep up hope for her recovery, but Wayne's sister, Evie, refused to accept platitudes—she wanted all the details. One afternoon when she called, Tammy was snoring softly on the bed. I thought surely she was asleep, so I said, "She has a slim to nil chance of beating this." Finally Evie understood.

When I hung up the phone, Tammy asked in a quiet, sad little voice, "Do I really have only a zero to nil chance?"

"No, honey," I said. "You have a slim to nil chance, not a zero to nil chance."

And it was true. She had an appointment with the doctors in Tucson the week after we were scheduled to return home to see if she could possibly get into the clinical trial for a new cancer drug. She did still have a slim chance to survive.

She had learned about some sort of herbal supplement that was supposed to help rebuild her immune system to better her chances for qualifying for the clinical trial. We found a store in Chicago that carried it, and even though it was obscenely expensive, we bought some. Unfortunately, when she took it, it was so nasty she barfed it up, along with everything she had eaten all day.

Small annoyances became major battles. First there was constipation, then diarrhea. And they all took their toll. She was so thin, so frail. It was as if a ghost walked in her shadow.

After her treatment regimen was finally finished, on August 29, we went home.

Tammy was the morphine queen for a while, but with the neutron treatments, her pain subsided dramatically, and she began to gradually come off the morphine.

One day we were going up the steps to her apartment, and the apartment manager was coming up the steps behind us. The bandage had slipped down on Tam's leg, exposing the large, gaping wound.

"Boy, that's going to leave a nasty scar, huh?" she said.

Tammy just laughed and said, "Yeah."

She finally accepted the fact that she was going to have to give up her apartment and move in with her dad and me. Giving up her independence was perhaps the hardest decision she had had to make so far. We paid the rent on her apartment for another month to give us plenty of time to make the move and for her to figure out what to do about her three cats.

Tam's wound, the incision that came apart, had to heal before she could take part in a clinical trial, but still we clung to the thread of hope that it would indeed heal soon.

-11-

$\mathcal{D}$uring a conversation with my friend Betty Peterson, I mentioned my dilemma about Tammy's cats—how to cope with three more cats in a house that already had a resident cat who thought he was master of the universe. Oscar was a long-haired orange cat that Tam had found as a tiny kitten, abandoned near her home when she was a graduate student at the University of New Mexico. Milo and Wiffle, who had been Terri's cats, were brothers and much younger and much larger than Oscar. When Betty asked if Tam would consider giving up some of her cats, I told her that Tam wouldn't like it, but that seemed to be the only solution. Betty promptly offered to take the two brothers. Her family's cat had recently died, and they had a huge two-story house with a basement, a perfect playhouse for cats.

Tammy reluctantly agreed to give up Milo and Wiffle. She insisted on going with me to deliver them to make sure their new home met with her approval. Betty showed her the area where the cat brothers would be free to roam, and it ranged from their own room on the top floor throughout the house, all the way down to the basement. Tam said good-bye to her cats as she turned them loose to explore their new home. But that wasn't really the end of them for her. Betty gave us frequent updates on their antics and adventures, which made the situation a bit easier for Tam.

She thought Oscar was too old and too attached to her to have to find a new home, and we agreed. Max, our cat, would just have to learn to share his home with Oscar.

Tam went through her things and chose what she wanted to bring with her to our house. She planned to bring her own bed, but we didn't have room for all her furniture and belongings in our house, so we rented a storage unit a couple of miles down the road to store the rest. It afforded her easy access to her things should she need them.

Wayne took her computer desk apart so we could get it downstairs, and Terri helped her pack the things she wanted to bring to our house. Cindy and her girls packed everything else. They labeled each box and stacked it in the living room of Tam's apartment. Once everything was packed, we began lugging furniture and boxes down the two flights of stairs and into our pickup. It took many trips and several days to get it all out.

Tam wanted to leave the apartment sparkling clean, but before we could even get started cleaning it, the apartment manager said there was absolutely no need. She had a cleaning crew ready to come in and take care of it; that was her gift to Tammy.

By mid-September, scans showed tumors growing in the lower lobes of both lungs and possibly one in her spleen. Still, she couldn't qualify for a clinical trial of an experimental drug because her split incision hadn't healed enough yet and her blood counts were still too low. Dr. Lobell suggested that she consider hyperbaric oxygen therapy to speed the healing process so she could qualify for the clinical trial.

Tammy did a bit of research to learn more about hyperbaric oxygen therapy (HBOT) and just where there might be facilities offering it close enough for her to access.

Hyperbaric oxygen chambers were developed to treat deep-sea divers who came from the high pressures of deep water up to the surface atmospheric pressure too soon and developed a painful and potentially fatal condition called the bends. A side benefit of the chambers is that they have also proven effective in accelerating the healing process. Tam learned that it is a legitimate treatment—Medicare even approves it.

There was a facility in Tucson, but they were booked and couldn't accept Tammy for treatment for several weeks. There was another one in El Paso, but there was one even closer to home, in Santa Fe, and they could begin her treatments immediately. That would be ideal. The drive from our home would only take an hour and a half or so each way; Tam could stay at home rather than in a hotel room.

Once again, her HMO threw up a roadblock. They would authorize Tam's treatment in Tucson but not in Santa Fe. Tam contested the decision, but they wouldn't budge. The HMO claimed that the doctor in Santa Fe wasn't yet board certified in hyperbaric medicine, only board eligible.

Terri came up with the idea of bartering her services for Tam's treatments.

She had had training in hyperbaric oxygen therapy treatment while she was working on her master's degree at the University of Miami. I think the offer impressed the people in Santa Fe. Dr. Ken Stoller, medical director of the Hyperbaric Medical Center, which was located in the same building as his pediatrics practice, thanked her very much for the offer but said that they would begin Tammy's treatments now and continue negotiating to get her HMO to pay for them.

The hyperbaric oxygen chamber was larger than I expected. It was shaped like a very large capsule with windows, and there was room inside for a dozen or so people to sit in comfort. One technician went inside with the patients while a team of technicians sat at a control center outside the chamber. They could see inside the chamber through the windows, and they communicated with those inside by microphone.

Before entering the chamber, people had to don all-cotton clothing and remove their shoes. If they wished, the group could choose a movie to watch from the facility's library, or they could listen to music or read. Once a session began, it took a while for the atmosphere inside the chamber to reach the proper pressure. Conversely, once it was finished, it took a while to return to the normal outside atmospheric pressure. Thus, unless there was some sort of emergency, once a session began, no one could leave the chamber until it was finished.

Each session lasted about two hours. To coax Tam's wound to heal as rapidly as possible, she had two treatments a day, from three to five days a week. The radiation burns on her neck and shoulder healed in just four days, and the dehisced wound began to fill in.

Cindy and Terri drove Tam to Santa Fe on their days off work, and I drove her the rest of the time, so it really wasn't an ordeal for any of us once we got the logistics worked out.

Wayne, Tammy, and I lived in Belen, about forty miles south of Albuquerque, and Albuquerque is about fifty-five miles south of Santa Fe. Fortunately, we could drive Interstate 25 most of the way, so it was a fairly easy trip. Tam had one treatment at 9:00 a.m. and the other at 1:00 p.m. generally, barring unforeseen circumstances. On the days when Cindy or Terri were taking her to Santa Fe, I drove her to the Cracker Barrel Restaurant parking lot beside the freeway in Albuquerque, where we met whoever was driving that day, and they drove the rest of the way and spent the day in Santa Fe. When they were ready to return to Albuquerque, they gave me a call by cell phone and I met them at the Cracker Barrel again and brought her home.

Either way, we tried to leave home by 7:00 a.m., and she was back by 5:00 p.m.

Tam thought she might feel a bit claustrophobic inside the chamber, but she didn't. She actually enjoyed her time in there. She said it was so peaceful; she could watch a movie or read or sleep if she wanted and forget about cancer for just a little while.

At first, we spent the time between the day's treatment sessions exploring Santa Fe. We browsed in the shops and walked through old neighborhoods. But as time went on, Tam just didn't have the energy for that anymore, so we found a shady spot in the nearby St. Vincent Hospital parking lot and chatted or listened to music on the car radio or napped.

To our good fortune, for one week in early October, our treks to Santa Fe coincided with the Albuquerque International Balloon Fiesta. Our timing was perfect that week. Each morning, we got to Albuquerque just as the balloons were lifting off or shortly thereafter, and the early morning sky filled with brightly colored hot-air balloons. Besides the round ones, the special-shaped balloons were flying too. There was a giant black-and-white cow balloon, one shaped like a castle, a huge, lumbering tractor-shaped one, a pink pig, Tony the Tiger, and many, many more.

The morning drives were truly magical that week, and though Tam was lying back on her seat, she loved watching the balloons in the bright blue morning sky.

While we were on the road, Wayne kept things in order at home as he had since our very first trip to Tucson so long ago. He kept up with the yard work, he shopped for groceries and supplies, he kept the house clean, and he paid the bills. Best of all, he fielded phone calls from worried relatives and friends and kept them updated on what was going on with Tam.

It became harder and harder for Tam to breathe, so Dr. Tarnower put her on oxygen. And she began to get two to three units of blood and one unit of platelets every week, then every three to four days.

By mid-October, her wound was still slowly filling, but the pain in her right leg and hip was getting more and more intense. She was using 125-milligram Duragesic pain patches and morphine tablets for breakthrough pain. She was so very miserable. At times, the morphine altered her personality and her disposition. Fragments of truth melded into a weird fantasy that became her truth.

On a Sunday we planned to take another road trip to Tucson to see if she would finally qualify for the elusive clinical trial. But the road trip never happened. Her very last option remained just out of reach. Her blood counts couldn't seem to get even remotely close to the minimum required for the clinical trial.

Little round blood-blister-looking bumps began to crop up on her torso, first just one under her left arm and then a few more here and there. When we showed them to Dr. Tarnower, she said they were caused by the cancer. I wanted to scream "No, they're not!" but she was the doctor, and she knew much more about these things than I did, so I said nothing. Still, I hoped there was a more innocuous explanation for them.

We put an ad in the newspaper to sell Tam's car. We had two calls, both of them from Santa Fe. One lady had totaled her car in an accident on the freeway just the week before. She wanted to see Tam's car but had no way to get to Belen to look at it. So the next day, Wayne drove Tam's car and followed us to the Hyperbaric Medical Center. While Tam had her treatment, the lady looked over Tam's car. She ended up paying cash for it and happily driving it away. Wayne and I spent the day just poking around Santa Fe while Tam had her treatments. It was a very nice day all around.

Dr. Tarnower suggested that Tam get a home health care nurse to come and check on her a couple of times a week and be sure her wound didn't get infected. The HMO paid for a nurse, and the nurse brought bandaging supplies with her so we didn't have to buy them anymore. That helped tremendously.

It finally dawned on me that it was time to get Tam's affairs in order. To provide help with her medical bills, we had to get her on disability before she was beyond disabled. We also had to close out her bank account, which proved to be a major hassle because she wasn't physically able to go to the bank and sit in the lobby for hours, waiting for someone to find the time to help her. But we got it done. Finally, I had to secure her medical power of attorney. We were extremely fortunate with that because there was a lawyer's office nearby, and she agreed to come to our house to do the paperwork.

Though Tammy had been really, really loopy that morning, when it was time for the lawyer to come, she pulled herself together and was perfectly coherent and lucid. She was bright and funny even. It must have taken tremendous effort, but she held on to lucidity the entire time the lawyer was at our house. Once the door closed behind her, Tammy made her way back to bed and slept for the rest of the day.

Snow! It was November 4, and already we were getting snow. Both Cindy and Terri called early in the morning to say it was snowing in Albuquerque. It wasn't yet snowing in Belen; however, it probably was in Santa Fe. Snow was a good excuse to stay home. But Tam insisted on going the next day, snow or not, even though it took every bit of energy she had just to get to the table to eat.

Tammy was still determined to get her HMO to pay for her hyperbaric oxygen treatments. So she summoned enough strength to write the following letter to the state, asking for an external review of her dispute with her HMO.

November 7, 2002

DEPARTMENT OF INSURANCE EXTERNAL REVIEW

I have metastatic angiosarcoma. In early May of this year, I had a tumor surgically excised from the back of my left thigh. Surgery was followed by brachytherapy (high-dose radiation delivered directly to the tumor bed). About four weeks after the surgery, the incision dehisced.

Since then, I have had more tumors, more chemotherapy, and more radiation, this time to my left shoulder, and the dehisced wound still has not healed.

I was referred to an oncologist at the University of Arizona Medical Center in Tucson who is familiar with my type of cancer. He has a clinical trial to offer me once this wound is healed. He recommended a minimum of six weeks of hyperbaric oxygen therapy (HBOT) to speed the healing process.

My HMO authorized HBOT treatment at the Tucson facility, but at this stage of my disease, the cost of travel and lodging make that an impossibility for both me and my family.

However, there is a facility in Santa Fe that provides hyperbaric oxygen therapy. It was recommended by people at the University of New Mexico Health Science Center and by the HBOT facility in El Paso, Texas.

My HMO has steadfastly refused to approve a referral for me to get treatment in Santa Fe, citing conflicting reasons.

-In a letter dated October 9 to Kathi Padilla of the Managed Health Care Bureau, Insurance Division, Dr. Mark Whitaker, vice president and medical director of my HMO stated that "Ms. Redman was not medically stable enough to receive the hyperbaric treatment."

- *In the conclusion portion of the October 24 Internal Medicine Panel Review report, Dr. Whitaker states that the review committee agrees that hyperbaric oxygen treatments are a covered benefit and are medically necessary and the requested treatment will be covered—in either Tucson or El Paso.*

-In the October 9 letter, Dr. Whitaker said, "There had been no requests, other than Ms. Redman's, for hyperbaric treatment in the past several years."

- *That's not quite true. In June 2002, my HMO approved six HBOT visits for one of their members to Dr. Ken Stoller, medical director of the Hyperbaric Medical Center of New Mexico in Santa Fe for hyperbaric oxygen therapy services. The authorization, on file in Dr. Stoller's office, approves "physician attendance and supervision."*

-Dr. Whitaker also said in the October 9 letter that "newer wound healing techniques, particularly the wound-vac system, have become more widely accepted for wound care than hyperbaric oxygen."

- *In his concluding statements of the Internal Medicine Panel Review, Dr. Whitaker says, "The Committee agrees hyperbaric oxygen treatments are a covered benefit and are medically necessary."*

-Finally, in the October 9 letter, Dr. Whitaker said that "if Dr. Stoller can demonstrate that he has met the training

requirements for Certification through the American Board of Medical Specialties in Hyperbaric Medicine, we will reconsider our denial of his request."

   •   *Phyllis Gaspin, certification reviewer with the American College of Hyperbaric Medicine responded. Dr. Stoller said that he expects to have completed the required 1,000 treatments and to earn his certification by the end of this year.*

   Dr. Stoller has a contract with my HMO for his pediatric practice, but his facility—the Hyperbaric Medical Center of New Mexico—does not. Dr. Stoller has stated that he is willing to work within the HMO guidelines without a contract in order to provide my treatment.

   If, according to Dr. Whitaker, my condition is unstable, how could traveling to Tucson or El Paso for six weeks, away from the support of my family and friends and incurring a debt that I cannot hope to pay, promote my healing and stabilize my condition?

   Though we both agree it's medically necessary, they will only approve this treatment at a facility unavailable to me, both financially and emotionally.

   I need my HMO's approval of my referral for treatment to heal my nonhealing wound so I can get into a clinical trial that might give me the chance to live.

Sincerely,
Tamara Redman

   It took them a long time to reach their decision, but ultimately, the external review board found in favor of Tammy's HMO. The Hyperbaric Medical Center received no payment for Tam's treatments there.

   As Tammy settled into her place inside the hyperbaric oxygen chamber on Friday, November 8, the technician put pillows behind her back and neck to try and make her comfortable. When it was time for her to come out of the chamber, the pillows behind her back were soaked with blood. One of the blood balloons on her back had started bleeding. The tech tried not to panic, but he was obviously worried. He put a pressure bandage on the oozing red bump and helped me get her to the car; she was so frail and weak she couldn't make it on her own. I laid the seat as far back as it would go, and he put pillows around her to make her as comfortable as possible and wished us a speedy and safe trip home. By the time we got home, the bleeding had stopped.

That was her last trip to Santa Fe.

-12-

$\mathcal{V}$ery early the next morning, the ominous red balloon began bleeding again, so I reapplied the pressure bandage. Soon one of the blood balloons under her arm began to bleed too, so I bandaged that one. But this time I could not get them to stop. They weren't gushing, but they wouldn't stop bleeding.

Our next-door neighbor Bernice Boyle was a retired army nurse, so when Tam's bleeding hadn't stopped by 8:30 a.m., I called and asked her to come over and help. But before I could ask her, Tam started vomiting blood—it gushed from her mouth like lava erupting from a volcano. I hung up on Bernice and ran to help Tam.

Bernice came right over and helped calm Tammy. By then the vomiting had stopped, but Tam was cold and clammy with beads of sweat on her forehead, and she was gasping for air. Bernice took her pulse and very calmly and quietly said that we needed to take her to the emergency room—*right now*!

We got to the emergency room at 9:24 a.m., and they mercifully put Tam in a private room on the emergency floor right away. Then the waiting began. It was hours before a doctor came to see her; she wasn't actually admitted to the hospital until 3:00 p.m.

She had a delightful, totally unexpected distraction, however, that made the wait much less traumatic for her.

At about 10:30 a.m., my cell phone rang and a male voice asked if I was Tammy Redman's mother. When I said yes, I was, he said he was an old friend of Tam's and he was out in the waiting room. It was Frank Roberts, who had been one of Tam's classmates at the University of Alabama in Birmingham. Frank and his wife, Lori, were Tammy's very good friends. Though they lived in Seattle these days, Frank had been to a conference and was passing through Albuquerque on his way back home. He had a couple of hours' layover in Albuquerque, so he tried to call Tam, but her phone had been disconnected. He knew we lived nearby, so he looked up our phone number in the local phone book. When he called our house, Wayne told him what was going on with Tam and gave him my cell phone number.

I went out to the waiting room to find him and led him back to Tam's room. She was so surprised and delighted to see him. She perked up and chatted almost as though her cancer ordeal was only a small inconvenience. He extended his stay until the next day so he could spend time with Tam.

I don't know where he found it, but to cheer her up, he brought her a tiny solar device that stuck to the window with a suction cup, and when the sun shined on it, a tiny prism slowly turned, casting little rainbows on the walls of the room as it turned. She loved it!

But she couldn't hold her good mood for long. By early afternoon, she was exhausted and grumpy, not with Frank but with Terri. It was as though she had a huge load of gripes and misery, and the only safe place to dump it was on Terri. Terri was her twin, after all, her alter ego, and Terri could and would help her carry this burden.

Tammy wasn't the only person being damaged by the monster that was cancer.

Several days later, Tammy finally agreed to go on hospice care but on her own terms. The goal—the function, really—of hospice is to make the patient as comfortable as possible while they wait to die. It is not to prolong life or to provide treatment to seek a cure. Thus they would provide oxygen but not—usually—such things as blood transfusions. Tammy agreed to accept hospice care but in the hospital, not at home. She was terrified of vomiting blood and of not being able to breathe again. We lived so far away, and it took so long to get to medical help. She was afraid to risk it. Also she insisted on continuing to receive the blood transfusions she so desperately needed. She finally convinced the doctors that the blood transfusions were necessary for her comfort; she wasn't trying to cheat death. It wasn't that she thought she could avoid dying; she just didn't want it to hurt. Amy Tarnower thought that was most reasonable, and Tam had her way.

Tam was moved to one of the two hospice rooms in the cancer ward. It was a private room big enough to accommodate visitors and family in comfort. Large windows on the west side of the room looked out over the city and to the west mesa beyond. All in all, it was a fairly nice place for Tam to spend her last days. The staff moved a recliner, a pillow, and extra blankets into the room, and Terri, Cindy, and I alternated spending the night with her, so she was never alone at night. Wayne or Cindy or Terri or I, or sometimes all of us, visited her during the day as well so someone would be there if she needed help. We tried to make life easier for the hospital staff, tending to Tam's care when we could by changing her bedsheets and bathing her and trying to keep her comfortable. They probably wouldn't have kicked us out anyway. They were very kind and considerate, but we wanted to make sure they would let us stay with Tam.

She seemed to be more aware of what was going on around her on this day. Her longtime friend Becky Rios just happened to call the day before. When she got the message saying Tam's phone had been disconnected, she called our house. She knew Tam had cancer, but she didn't know that Tam had become so much sicker. When I arrived at Tam's room Thursday morning, there was Becky. She had flown in that morning from San Antonio, Texas. She stayed at a hotel within walking distance of the hospital, and the only time she left Tam's room was to eat and to return to her hotel room for the night. The two had been roommates while Tammy was in graduate school at the University of New Mexico. When Tam was lucid, they talked about old times and just girl talk. When Tam slept or hallucinated, Becky just sat with her. While she was there, Becky ordered a huge arrangement of stargazer lilies to be delivered to Tam's room. To Tam's enormous joy, Becky stayed several days before she flew back to her home in Texas.

On Monday, November 18, Gail came to spend a week. She spent the nights with Terri and spent the days with Tam. On Tuesday, yet another friend from Tam's grad school days in Birmingham flew in to see her. Cecily Harmon and her family lived in Florida, but Cecily took time off from her work to fly to Albuquerque and spend a few days with Tammy.

Tammy was both delighted and surprised by the visits. She certainly couldn't say that nobody cared.

I too was pleased that these lovely people had interrupted their lives to come and offer their love and comfort to Tam. But I found myself feeling a bit disgruntled. I got angry for no reason at all. Looking back now, I think a part of me resented having to share Tam's last days with someone else. It's not something I'm proud of, but I couldn't help it.

I don't know if it was the pain medications or the disease, but Tammy had retreated into her own world, a place that existed in fragments in her mind. For three days in a row, though, she was awake and aware of what was going on around her. When Dr. Stoller from the Hyperbaric Medical Center made one of his regular calls to check on Tam, I told him she seemed to be doing much better.

"I hate to tell you this," he said, "but in my practice and from what other docs have said, people tend to get their act together just before they cross over."

Gradually, Tam slipped back into mostly sleep and hallucination.

Nearly every day, some of Tam's friends came to visit, and most of them brought flowers. My friend Eloisa sent her a bouquet of sunflowers, Tammy's favorite flowers because they are bold and cheerful and tough. She got roses and daisies, all kinds of flowers. Dave Bice and his wife came several times. Once they brought a bouquet of flowers arranged in a delightful little teacup and saucer.

I don't know where she got the idea, but once the flowers started to fade, Terri took them home and let them dry out completely, then she pulled off the petals and layered them in a tall apothecary jar with a bit of salt to keep them dry. She kept the jar on the shelf across from Tam's bed so Tam could see all the flowers she had received. Even when Tam seemed unaware of what was going on around her, she seemed to need to see that apothecary jar filled with dry flower petals.

Richard was—and is—an artist, among other things. Tammy especially loved his abstract drawings. So when he came to see her the first time, he brought one to put up on the wall across from her bed where she could see it. She was so pleased. He brought a different one to exchange each time he came to visit, which was nearly every day. When he came to visit her, Cindy or Terri or Wayne or I chatted with him for a while, then left to have a cup of coffee or to go for a stroll so they could have some time alone.

On Monday, November 25, Tammy was wide awake and very much aware when I got to her room.

"Isn't there something out there for me? Are you sure there isn't a clinical trial somewhere? I don't mind traveling, I can do it."

"No, hon, there's nothing left. Your cancer is just too pervasive." I was her very last thread of hope, and I had to crush her one last effort to live.

"It's okay. I hate it, but it's okay."

"Am I going to die today?"

"I'm so tired, I don't want to be sick anymore."

"I'm scared. I want to see Daddy and Terri and Cindy."

It had been about two weeks since I had seen Dr. Tarnower in the hall and asked her how much time she thought Tammy had left. She said about two weeks probably, maybe a little more because she was young and had a strong heart.

Death hovered in the corners of Tam's room.

That night, the hospital staff lugged in three more recliners along with pillows and blankets. Terri, Cindy, Wayne, and I all spent the night with Tam in her room. Terri pulled her recliner next to Tam's bed and held her hand all night long as if she could hold her back should death come for her in the night.

Tammy had gotten two units of blood on Wednesday and another two on Thanksgiving morning. All day long, she was awake, aware, and alert. Propped up on a bank of pillows, she held court for the many friends who came to visit her. I had spent the night with her, and Wayne came at about 11:00 a.m. Terri and Mark joined us at about 12:30 p.m. Cindy cooked a full-fledged Thanksgiving dinner—turkey, dressing, the works—and brought it to us at the hospital that afternoon. Heather and Chelsea came with her to see Tam and to help Cindy haul the food up to the hospital's fourth-floor lounge, where they filled our plates and brought them to us in Tam's room. The food was scrumptious, but I wasn't hungry.

We ate at about 4:00 p.m. After everyone had finished and chatted a while, Cindy and her girls packed everything up and hauled it back down to their car. Cindy took Heather and Chelsea home, then came back to spend the night with Tam.

Tam's back started to hurt, so a nurse gave her a morphine injection, and finally, after going all day without so much as a nap, she went to sleep, and Wayne and I went home.

Friday night was my turn to stay with Tam. Vicky, the hospice nurse, came by and said they were going to release Tam to go home Tuesday if things continued to go as well as they had so far. Later Dr. Tarnower came by to see how Tam was doing, and I asked her about Tam's possible release from the hospital. Yes, she said, they were thinking about sending her home Tuesday, but they would see how the weekend went and take things one day at a time. I welcomed the idea of her coming home, but I wasn't sure she was strong enough. Besides, her original reasons for wanting to stay in the hospital were still valid. I didn't think she would make it till Thanksgiving, but she did. As one of her friends who also had terminal cancer had said, every day was a gift.

Her condition was subtly changing. She didn't seem to be bleeding so much anymore. She didn't wake up with blood caked on her teeth and lips, and the tiny blood balloon on her back wasn't oozing blood anymore. But she was having pain in her abdomen and back. She needed more pain medication, and between that and fatigue from the Thanksgiving festivities, she slept most of the day. Nevertheless, it was another gift.

On Sunday, Tammy slept most of the day, and another of her blood balloons—this time on her shoulder—began oozing. She had received more blood and platelets earlier in the day. It was my turn to spend the night with her again. As I watched her sleep, it broke my heart. She was there; her essence, her spirit, and her soul were there. How could she die? How could it all just cease to exist? How could I possibly let her go? As If I had a choice.

My world had gotten smaller and smaller and smaller until it encompassed only Tam's hospital room, our house, and the road between. I had, gradually but almost completely, cut off outside connections—my job, organizations to which I belonged, all but my closest friends. It hadn't been so long ago that I was worried about keeping all the balls in the air, keeping up with all the obligations and expectations that life gave me. Now all the balls had come crashing down, and I didn't even care.

Dave Bice has many talents. Besides being a research scientist and a pilot, he plays the cello. On Monday afternoon, December 2, he and one of his friends brought their cellos to give Tammy her own private concert. They played the Sonate I Prelude by Joseph Bodin de Boismortier and several of James Hook's cello duets, among other compositions.

Dick Fate and his wife, Suzanne, and her son were in the room, visiting Tam. She was awake and alert, enjoying her guests. We shut the door to her room so we wouldn't disturb other patients, and Dave Bice and his friend made the loveliest music ever. It was as if we had front-row seats in a concert hall, and actually, I suppose we did. Tammy was absolutely enchanted. It was the best concert ever for her, a priceless gift.

When they were finished, they carefully opened the door, and a cluster of staff and patients scattered. They too had been enjoying the concert.

Later, Dave Bice told me that he had played on a brand-new cello that day, one that he made himself. Actually, it wasn't quite finished—it hadn't yet been varnished. And since each cello has its own name, that one is named Tammy.

Monday was her last fully lucid day.

Tammy still clung to life on Friday. The hospice people had decided against discharging her to go home. Tuesday night and Wednesday, Tammy had a really rough time, pulling off her oxygen mask and trying to get the hell out of there—she was done with the cancer thing; she wanted to go home. Meanwhile, she was vomiting blood profusely.

Soon after Thanksgiving, she began sliding downhill, and Dr. Tarnower had put her on a Decadron drip, a steroid concoction administered intravenously to boost the effect of the pain and antinausea medication while boosting Tam's appetite and feelings of well-being and keeping her blood pressure up in the normal range. It worked for about a week. But one of the side effects was a feeling of edginess, which probably accounted for her being determined to rip off all restraints and go home. Since Tammy was no longer lucid and could no longer benefit from the Decadron drip, with our permission, Dr. Tarnower discontinued it and put her on a morphine drip so she wouldn't feel pain. The doctor said that within six to twenty-four hours, Tam's blood pressure would plummet and her heart would stop beating. Soon after the Decadron drip was stopped, Tam started gasping for air even though she was on oxygen, and her body curled to the left. The nurse said that was the "fish out of water" breathing pattern, a precursor to death. So Terri and Cindy came over from work, and Wayne drove our old pickup in, and we stayed with her all day and all night.

Twenty-four hours later, she was still breathing. Her gasping was much gentler, and her eyes were rolled back, either in a coma or a very deep sleep. Terri insisted that it was because she was being her usual slow, methodical self, and she wanted to be sure she did this thing right. By Wednesday and Thursday, we were the Kleenex Brigade, but by Friday, we were making dumb jokes. We just knew that Tammy was aware of our antics and would have cracked a few dumb jokes of her own if she could have. I had been at the hospital for three nights in a row, so I went home to shower and change clothes. Everybody left for a few hours, except Terri. She told Tam that she was going to wait her out; she was not going away, so Tam could take as long as she wanted.

Tammy lost her battle with cancer at 1:08 p.m. on Saturday, December 7. In typical Tammy fashion, she was a slowpoke, living on for fifty hours after Dr. Tarnower said she would last only six to twenty-four hours at the most. Her lungs were completely filled with tumor, and her breathing stopped—but not her heart. Refusing to give up, it kept beating for over five more minutes.

It's strange how your priorities change. It had seemed like just yesterday that I had prayed to God begging him to let her live, and then I was praying for him to let her die. Yet I still wasn't ready to let her go. Terri and I were with her, as were two of Terri's and Tam's very good friends, Chris Glidden and her daughter, Jenna. We were making plans for a 10K and 5K run on New Year's Day to be held in Tam's honor, to raise money to help cancer patients pay for the necessities that insurance doesn't cover. Terri and Chris had talked to Tammy about it several months earlier, and she was both honored and delighted with the idea of the run.

As we talked, Tam just stopped breathing. Her ordeal was finally over.

By the time she died, her hair was about an inch long and curled around the oxygen tube that looped over her ears; her dehisced wound was almost completely healed.

-13-

We held Tammy's memorial service at the First Unitarian Church in Albuquerque on Friday, December 13. Tammy would have loved the irony, having her service on Friday the 13th. She wanted to be cremated; she did not want people staring at her remains without her there to defend herself, so that's what we did.

After we had explored several possible sites for Tam's service and just couldn't find what we wanted, Cindy had suggested the First Unitarian Church. It had lots of windows, lots of light, and lots of room, yet it wasn't too big and it was affordable. It was as nearly perfect as we could find.

Chris and Jenna Glidden took some of our photos of Tam, enlarged them, and mounted them in a series of collages on display boards. They enlarged a portrait of Tam to 18" × 24", then mounted and framed it. We put that on top of the piano on the stage and framed it with an L-shaped arrangement of red roses and pine boughs. Then we displayed the collages on a long table and put more pine boughs and long-stemmed red roses in front of them. Two large poinsettia plants framed the podium, with smaller ones along the front of the stage. Tam would have liked it, I think. It was very simple but elegant.

Fabian Gagnon, the chaplain at the hospital where Tam died, led the service. Tam had worked with him when she volunteered at the hospital after her first bout with this cancer, and she had had several long talks with him during her last days. When he agreed to do the service, he asked what sort of service we wanted. We told him we wanted to concentrate on celebrating her life, and that's what he did.

Just before the service began, Sue Michalik drove up in a taxi. Tam had worked under her as a postdoctoral fellow in Birmingham. Sue had flown in from Birmingham that morning and had taken the taxi directly to the church. We invited her to sit with us in the family section. The church was packed with Tam's friends and family.

We asked the soundman who worked at the church to take care of the microphones and the music for the service, and he did a beautiful job. We requested Beethoven's "Ode to Joy," Raspigi's "Pines of Rome," and a Hawaiian version of "Somewhere Over the Rainbow." He chose the rest of the background music.

I was astonished by how many people had something to say about Tammy when Chaplain Gagnon asked for comments. One of my favorites was when Dr. Lewis Nemes, her counselor, said that she was a closet genius and that she was a warrior who fought the good fight to the very end.

Next to all the warm, funny, comforting comments by Tammy's friends, the best part of the service was the music played by Cindy's friend Jeremy Marley on his violin. He chose most of his own music, but we asked him to play "Amazing Grace" as the finale. The music coming from his violin as he played this song sounded like it was being played on bagpipes. Nearly every one of the 125 or so people there was moved to tears.

After the service, most of Tam's friends lingered to chat a while, then left, but family members made the hour-long drive to our house in Belen. Cousins and aunts and uncles and my mother, Tam's only living grandmother, had come from as far as Arizona and California. My memory of the logistics of getting the house in order and providing food is a blur, but Wayne's cousin, Dick Frazier, and his wife, Sherron, took care of the details, making sure everything was in order. The thing I do remember is all the family members, from my side and from Wayne's side, talking and enjoying each other's company. From my perspective, it was a priceless moment in time when everyone was comfortable and kind and gentle. No one was left to sit in a corner ignored. Wayne kept an eye on my eighty-nine-year-old mother, getting her refreshments and carrying on a lively conversation with her. People talked and laughed and enjoyed the camaraderie. Tam would have loved that.

Early on, I read Elizabeth Kubler Ross's book on death and dying. In it, Kubler Ross said that if she had a choice, she would choose to die of cancer. I thought that was appalling! No one in their right mind would choose the pain and prolonged sense of doom that comes with a diagnosis of terminal cancer. I would much prefer a quick death, preferably in my sleep. But in retrospect, I can see some advantages for Tammy. Before the last few months of her life, she had no idea that so many people truly loved her. She had no idea how tough she really was or how much she could endure.

During that last year when we spent so much time on the road, I got to really, truly know her as a traveling companion, as a person, and as a friend. And I saw just how strong and how loving our family was. Tammy gave us all memories that we will treasure forever. She taught us the value of being alive.

Epilogue

$\mathcal{J}$ust before Christmas after Tam died, I was driving down NM47 toward the town of Los Lunas to do some very last-minute shopping at Staples and Walgreens. It was only a little after five, but already the sun had gone down and the sky was washed with pink and coral light. I looked up and saw a string of sandhill cranes flying over, headed for the river to bed down for the night. The cranes migrate to the Rio Grande valley in central New Mexico to spend the winter. Then there were more and more strands of cranes—hundreds, thousands of cranes. It almost looked as if the sky was covered with a huge net, and the net was made of flying cranes—a dark net against a coral-colored sky.

I glanced to the east, and a huge yellow full moon was rising from behind the mountains. It was a magical moment of beauty that I may never see again. Ordinary things juxtaposed in perfect harmony for just that one instant.

Tears trickled down my cheek and then progressed to deep sobs. There were so many things Tammy wanted to cram into the short time she had left. So many things to do and to see. One by one she had to give them up, but the one thing she really wanted was to see the cranes just one more time.

It was not to be; the cancer grew too fast.

Winter

the wind howls and sweeps in a sheet
along the edge of the freeway
grass and litter and blows into the sky
rising up higher than the car here below
on a side road
it rises and catches light
looking for a moment like magic dust

insolent clouds dip low and hang a heavy gray
they spit white bits of snow
that get taken up by the wind and whirl
around
whirl around and up out of sight

winter comes in and dances
on cold ground and black asphalt
the car shivers at a red stoplight
and holds back just an instant when trying to go east
against the wind pushing hard

my friend lost her daughter yesterday

she fought as hard as the wind pushes this sad morning
fought and pushed back the rampant cells that tried for
so long

to overtake her

she kicked them again and again

sick and weak, she flailed against the onslaught

winning at times

losing ground

but fighting every step and breath of the way

her ordeal is over

said my friend

I don't know if mine ever will be

I pray the wind has taken her up

whirling her around letting her see the wide and grand vistas

of life's design

taking her higher than this cold

sad

hardened earth

where pain can no longer find her

where her burden has blown away

delivering her into a place that is soft

and radiantly warm

This poem was written by my friend Sandy Starr soon after Tammy died. She was the one who first searched the Internet for information about angiosarcoma and learned about neutron radiation and the Fermilab. She passed the information on to Tam. Sandy was diagnosed with liver cancer a year or so after Tammy's death and died in 2005.